Surgery at a Glance

Surgery at a Glance

Pierce Grace

MCh, FRCSI, FRCS
Professor of Surgical Science
University of Limerick Graduate Medical School
Midwestern Regional Hospital
Limerick

Neil R. Borley

FRCS, FRCS (Ed), MS
Consultant Colorectal Surgeon
Cheltenham General Hospital
Cheltenham

Fourth edition

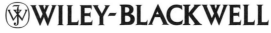

A John Wiley & Sons, Ltd., Publication

This edition first published 2009, © 2009 by Pierce Grace and Neil R. Borley
Previous editions: 1999, 2002, 2006

Blackwell Publishing was acquired by John Wiley & Sons in February 2007. Blackwell's publishing program has been merged with Wiley's global Scientific, Technical and Medical business to form Wiley-Blackwell.

Registered office: John Wiley & Sons Ltd, The Atrium, Southern Gate, Chichester, West Sussex, PO19 8SQ, UK

Editorial offices: 9600 Garsington Road, Oxford, OX4 2DQ, UK
The Atrium, Southern Gate, Chichester, West Sussex, PO19 8SQ, UK
111 River Street, Hoboken, NJ 07030-5774, USA

For details of our global editorial offices, for customer services and for information about how to apply for permission to reuse the copyright material in this book please see our website at www.wiley.com/wiley-blackwell

The right of the authors to be identified as the authors of this work has been asserted in accordance with the Copyright, Designs and Patents Act 1988.

Wiley also publishes its books in a variety of electronic formats. Some content that appears in print may not be available in electronic books.

Designations used by companies to distinguish their products are often claimed as trademarks. All brand names and product names used in this book are trade names, service marks, trademarks or registered trademarks of their respective owners. The publisher is not associated with any product or vendor mentioned in this book. This publication is designed to provide accurate and authoritative information in regard to the subject matter covered. It is sold on the understanding that the publisher is not engaged in rendering professional services. If professional advice or other expert assistance is required, the services of a competent professional should be sought.

Library of Congress Cataloging-in-Publication Data
Grace, P. A. (Pierce A.)
    Surgery at a glance / Pierce Grace, Neil R. Borley. — 4th ed.
      p.; cm. — (At a glance series)
    Includes index.
    ISBN 978-1-4051-8325-3
    1. Diagnosis, Surgical—Handbooks, manuals, etc.   2. Operations, Surgical—Handbooks, manuals, etc.   3. Surgery—Handbooks, manuals, etc.   I. Borley, Neil R.   II. Title.   III. Series: At a glance series (Oxford, England)
    [DNLM: 1. Surgical Procedures, Operative—Handbooks.   2. Diagnostic Techniques and Procedures—Handbooks. WO 39 G729c 2009]
    RD35.G68 2009
    617′.9—dc22

                                                                                        2009009669

ISBN: 978-1-4051-8325-3

A catalogue record for this book is available from the British Library.

Set in 9.5/12pt Times by Graphicraft Limited, Hong Kong
Printed and bound in Singapore

1   2009

Contents

Preface

Since its first publication in 1999 *Surgery at a Glance* has become a firm favourite with medical students and others who study surgery. Apart from the easy-to-use layout of the book, which is in keeping with the general style of the *At a Glance* series, one of its best features is its division into clinical presentations and surgical diseases. Thus, in one volume is combined the variety of ways that patients present with surgical problems and the surgical diseases that produce those presentations. Ten years on we are delighted to present the revised and updated fourth edition of *Surgery at a Glance*.

The new edition contains some significant improvements. Over the years the book has become more colourful with increasing amounts of colour being added to each new edition. In the fourth edition we have employed full colour throughout the text, which transforms the look of the book and makes it much easier to use. The 'Key points' and 'Key investigations' sections of the text are easily read and the colour illustrations are magnificent. A complete revision of the chapters and updating of the text for the fourth edition has resulted in some changes, but without an increase in the size of the book. 'Haematemesis' and 'Rectal bleeding' have been merged into a new chapter entitled 'Gastrointestinal bleeding'. A new chapter on 'Sepsis' has been added which complements the chapters on 'SIRS' and 'Surgical infection'; 'Paediatric general surgery' has been revised to conform to the general style of the book.

We have had lots of help and suggestions from several people in putting this book together. We would like to thank the many medical students and colleagues who have read the book and given us good advice. Students seem to like this book particularly for revision in preparation for exams. We especially thank the publishing team and illustrators at Wiley-Blackwell Publishing for their hard work in bringing this beautifully presented book to completion. We believe that the fourth edition of *Surgery at a Glance* is the best yet and we hope that this text will continue to help students understand surgery.

Pierce Grace
Neil R. Borley
2009

List of abbreviations

AAA	abdominal aortic aneurysm
AAT	aspartate amino transferase
ABI	ankle–brachial pressure index
Abs	antibiotics
ACE	angiotensin converting enzyme
Ach	acetylcholine
ACN	acute cortical necrosis
ACTH	adrenocorticotrophic hormone
ADH	antidiuretic hormone
AF	atrial fibrillation
AFP	α-fetoprotein
Ag	antigen
AKI	acute kidney injury
Alb	albumin
ALI	acute lung injury
ANCA	antineutrophil cytoplasmic antibody
ANDI	abnormalities of the normal development and involution (of the breast)
AP	angina pectoris
AP	anteroposterior
APACHE	acute physiology and chronic health evaluation
APTT	activated partial thromboplastin time
ARDS	adult/acute respiratory distress syndrome
ARF	acute renal failure
ASA	American Society of Anesthesiologists
ATN	acute tubular necrosis
AV	arteriovenous
BCC	basal cell carcinoma
BCG	bacillus Calmette–Guérin
BE	base excess
BEP	bleomycin, etoposide, cisplatin
BMI	body mass index
BP	blood pressure
BPH	benign prostatic hypertrophy
BS	breath sounds
C&S	culture and sensitivity
CABG	coronary artery bypass graft
CAD	coronary artery disease
cAMP	cyclic adenosine monophosphate
CA-MRSA	community-associated methicillin-resistant *Staphylococcus aureus*
CAS	carotid angioplasty and stent
CBD	common bile duct
CCF	congestive cardiac failure
CD	*Clostridium difficile*
CDI	central diabetes insipidus
CEA	carcinoembryonic antigen
CEA	carotid endarterectomy
cfu	colony forming units
CK	creatinine kinase
CLO	*Campylobacter*-like organism
CMV	cisplatin, methotrexate, vinblastine
CMV	cytomegalovirus

CNS	central nervous system
COCP	combined oral contraceptive pill
COPD	chronic obstructive pulmonary disease
COX	cyclo-oxygenase
CPK-MB	creatine phosphokinase (cardiac type)
CRC	colorectal carcinoma
CRF	chronic renal failure
CRP	C-reactive protein
CSF	cerebrospinal fluid
CT	computed tomography
CTA	computed tomographic angiogram
CVA	cerebrovascular accident
CVI	chronic venous insufficiency
CVP	central venous pressure
CVS	cardiovascular system
CXR	chest X-ray
D_2	type 2 dopaminergic receptors
DHEA	dihydroepiandrosterone
DIC	disseminated intravascular coagulation
DM	diabetes mellitus
DMSA	dimercaptosuccinic acid
DU	duodenal ulcer
DVT	deep venous thrombosis
Dx	diagnosis
DXA	dual energy X-ray absorptiometry
DXT	deep X-ray therapy
EAS	external anal sphincter
EBV	Epstein–Barr virus
ECG	electrocardiogram
EMLA	Eutetic Mixture of Local Anaesthetic
ER	oestrogen receptor
ERCP	endoscopic retrograde cholangio-pancreatograph
ESR	erythrocyte sedimentation rate
ESWL	extracorporeal shock-wave lithotripsy
EUA	examination under anaesthesia
EUS	endoscopic ultrasound
FBC	full blood count
FCD	fibrocystic disease
FFP	fresh frozen plasma
FHx	family history
FNAC	fine-needle aspiration cytology
FOB	faecal occult blood
FSH	follicle-stimulating hormone
5-FU	5-fluorouracil
γ-GT	gamma glutamyl transpeptidase
GA	general anaesthetic
GC	gemcitabine, cisplatin
GCS	Glasgow Coma Scale
GFR	glomerular filtration rate
GH	growth hormone
GI	gastrointestinal
Gm+, Gm−	Gram-positive, Gram-negative

GORD	gastro-oesophageal reflux disease	**MAG3**	mercapto acetyl triglycine
GSF	greater sciatica foramen	**MAP**	mean arterial pressure
GTN	glyceryl trinitrate	**MC+S**	microscopy cultures and sensitivity
GU	gastric ulcer	**MDRO**	multidrug-resistant organisms
GU	genito-urinary	**MDT**	multidisciplinary team
GVHD	graft-versus-host disease	**MEAC**	minimum effective analgesic concentration
Hb	haemoglobin	**MEN**	multiple endocrine neoplasia
β-HCG	β-human chorionic gonadotrophin	**MI**	myocardial infarction
HCG	human chorionic gonadotrophin	**MIBG**	*meta*-iodo-benzyl guanidine
Hct	haematocrit	**MM**	malignant melanoma
HDL	high density lipoprotein	**MND**	motor neurone disease
HDU	high-dependency unit	**MODS**	multiple organ dysfunction syndrome
HER2/neu	Human epidermal growth factor receptor 2	**MRA**	magnetic resonance angiography
HIDA	hepatabiliary imido-diacetic acid	**MRCP**	magnetic resonance cholangio-pancreatography
HLA	human leucocyte antigen	**MRI**	magnetic resonance imaging
HNPCC	hereditary non-polyposis colorectal cancer	**MRSA**	methicillin-resistant *Staphylococcus aureus*
HVA	homovanillic acid	**MS**	multiple sclerosis
Hx	history	**MSH**	melanocyte-stimulating hormone
IBS	irritable bowel syndrome	**MSU**	mid-stream urine
ICP	intracranial pressure	**MT**	major trauma
ICS	intercostal space	**MTP**	metatarsophalangeal
ICU	intensive care unit	**MUGA**	multiple uptake gated analysis
Ig	immunoglobulin	**MVAC**	methotrexate, vinblastine, doxorubicin
IGF	insulin-like growth factor		(Adriamycin), cisplatin
IL	interleukin	**N&V**	nausea and vomiting
iNOS	inducible nitric oxide synthetase	**NAdr**	noradrenaline/norepinephrine
INR	international normalized ratio	**NDI**	nephrogenic diabetes insipidus
IPPV	intermittent positive pressure ventilation	**NSAID**	non-steroidal anti-inflammatory drug
IV	intravenous	**NSGCT**	non-seminomatous germ cell tumour
IVC	inferior vena cava	**NSU**	non-specific urethritis
IVU	intravenous urogram	**OA**	osteoarthritis
JGA	juxtaglomerular apparatus	**o/e**	on examination
JVP	jugular venous pulse	**OGD**	oesophago-gastro-duodenoscopy
KUB	kidney, ureter, bladder	**OGJ**	oesophago-gastric junction
LA	local anaesthetic	**PA**	posteroanterior
LAD	left anterior descending	**PAD**	peripheral arterial disease
LATS	long-acting thyroid stimulating (factor)	**PAF**	platelet activating factor
LCA	left coronary artery	**PCA**	patient-controlled analgesia
LDH	lactate dehydrogenase	**PCV**	packed cell volume
LDL	low density lipoprotein	**PE**	pulmonary embolism
LDUH	low dose unfractionated heparin	**PEG**	percutaneous endoscopic gastrostomy
LFT	liver function test	**PEEP**	positive end expiratory pressure
LH	luteinizing hormone	**PET**	positron emission tomography
LHRH	LH-releasing hormone	**PID**	pelvic inflammatory disease
LIF	left iliac fossa	**PL**	prolactin
LMWH	low molecular weight heparin	**POP**	plaster of Paris
LOC	loss of consciousness	**POVD**	peripheral occlusive vascular disease
LOS	lower oesophageal sphincter	**PPI**	proton pump inhibitor
LPS	lipopolysaccharide	**PR**	per rectum
LRD	living related donor	**PSA**	prostate-specific antigen
LSE	left sternal edge	**PT**	prothrombin time
LSF	lesser sciatica foramen	**PTH**	parathyroid hormone
LSV	long saphenous vein	**PUD**	peptic ulcer disease
LUQ	left upper quadrant	**PUO**	pyrexia of unknown origin
LURD	living unrelated donor	**PV**	per vaginum
LV	left ventricle	**PVD**	peripheral vascular disease
LVF	left ventricular failure	**QoL**	quality of life

RBC	red blood cell
RCC	renal cell carcinoma
RD	respiratory depression
rhAPC	recombinant human activated protein C
RIA	radioimmunoassay
RIF	right iliac fossa
RLN	recurrent laryngeal nerve
RPLND	retroperitoneal lymph node dissection
RS	respiratory system
RT	radiotherapy
RTA	road traffic accident
RUQ	right upper quadrant
RV	right ventricle
RVF	right ventricular failure
Rx	treatment
SCC	squamous cell carcinoma
SGCT	seminomatous germ cell tumour
SIADH	syndrome of inappropriate antidiuretic hormone
SIRS	systemic inflammatory response syndrome
SLE	systemic lupus erythematosus
SLN	superior laryngeal nerve
SRS	somatostatin receptor scintigraphy
SSV	short saphenous vein
SVC	superior vena cava
T$_3$	tri-iodothyronine
T$_4$	thyroxine
TB	tuberculosis
TCC	transitional cell carcinoma

TED	thrombo-embolic deterrent
TENS	transcutaneous electrical nerve stimulation
TIA	transient ischaemic attack
TNF	tumour necrosis factor
TNM	tumour, node, metastasis (UICC)
tPA	tissue plasminogen activator
TPHA	treponema pallidum haemagglutination (test)
TPR	temperature, pulse, respiration
TRUS	transrectal ultrasound
TSH	thyroid-stimulating hormone
TURP	transurethral resection of the prostate
TURT	transurethral resection of tumour
UC	ulcerative colitis
UDT	undescended testis
U+E	urea and electrolytes
UI	urinary incontinence
U/S	ultrasound
UTI	urinary tract infection
VF	ventricular fibrillation
VHL	von Hippel–Lindau
VIP	vasoactive intestinal peptide
VMA	vanillyl mandelic acid
V/Q	ventilation–perfusion
VRE	vancomycin-resistant enterococcus
VSD	ventricular septal defect
WBC	white blood cell
WCC	white cell count

1 Neck lump

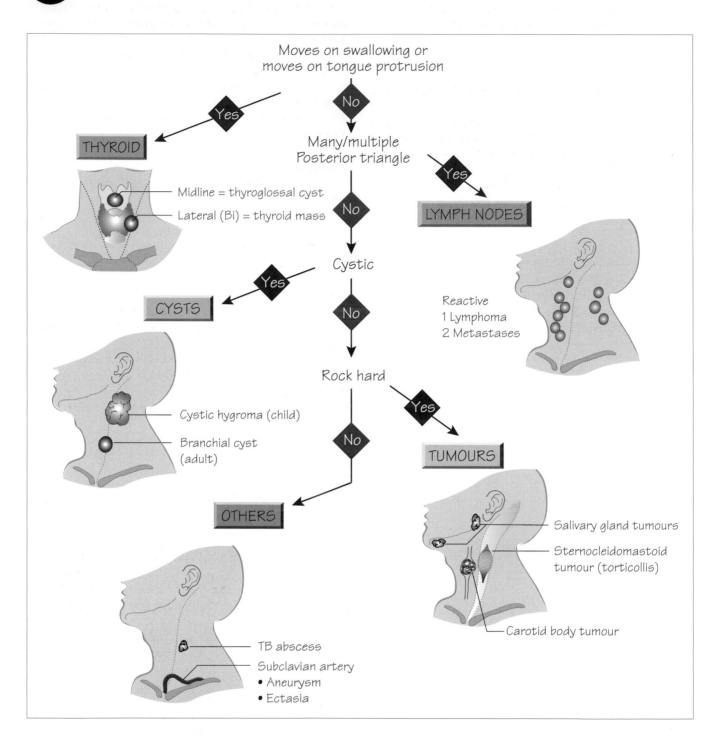

Moves on swallowing or
moves on tongue protrusion

No → Many/multiple Posterior triangle

Yes → THYROID

Midline = thyroglossal cyst
Lateral (Bi) = thyroid mass

Yes → LYMPH NODES

Reactive
1 Lymphoma
2 Metastases

No → Cystic

Yes → CYSTS

Cystic hygroma (child)
Branchial cyst (adult)

No → Rock hard

Yes → TUMOURS

Salivary gland tumours
Sternocleidomastoid tumour (torticollis)
Carotid body tumour

No → OTHERS

TB abscess
Subclavian artery
• Aneurysm
• Ectasia

 Surgery at a Glance, 4e. By P. Grace and N.R. Borley. Published 2009 by Blackwell Publishing. ISBN 978-1-4051-8325-3.

Definition

A *neck lump* is any congenital or acquired mass arising in the anterior or posterior triangles of the neck between the clavicles inferiorly and the mandible and base of the skull superiorly.

> ### Key points
>
> • Thyroid swellings move upwards (with the trachea) on swallowing.
> • Most abnormalities of the neck are visible as swellings.
> • Ventral lumps attached to the hyoid bone, such as thyroglossal cysts, move upwards with both swallowing and protrusion of the tongue.
> • Multiple lumps are almost always lymph nodes.
> • Don't forget a full head and neck examination, including the oral cavity, in all cases of lymphadenopathy.

Differential diagnosis

• 50% of neck lumps are thyroid in origin.
• 40% of neck lumps are caused by malignancy (80% metastatic usually from primary lesion above the clavicle; 20% primary neoplasms: lymphomas, salivary gland tumours).
• 10% of neck lumps are inflammatory or congenital in origin.

Thyroid

• Goitre, cyst, neoplasm.

Neoplasm

• Metastatic carcinoma.
• Primary lymphoma.
• Salivary gland tumour.
• Sternocleidomastoid tumour.
• Carotid body tumour (rare).

Inflammatory

• Acute infective adenopathy.
• Collar stud abscess.
• Parotitis.

Congenital

• Thyroglossal duct cyst.
• Dermoid cyst.
• Torticollis.
• Branchial cyst.
• Cystic hygroma.

Vascular

• Subclavian or brachiocephalic ectasia (common).
• Subclavian aneurysm (rare).

Important diagnostic features
Children

• Congenital and inflammatory lesions are common.
• Cystic hygroma: in infants, base of the neck, brilliant transillumination, 'come and go'.

• Thyroglossal or dermoid cyst: midline, discrete, elevates with tongue protrusion.
• Torticollis: rock hard mass, more prominent with head flexed, associated with fixed rotation (a fibrous mass in the sternocleidomastoid muscle).
• Branchial cyst (also fistulae or sinus): anterior to the upper third of the sternocleidomastoid.
• Viral/bacterial adenitis: usually affects jugular nodes, multiple, tender masses.
• Neoplasms are unusual in children (lymphoma most common).

Young adults

Inflammatory neck masses and thyroid malignancy are common.
• Viral (e.g. infectious mononucleosis) or bacterial (tonsillitis/pharyngitis) adenitis.
• Papillary thyroid cancer: isolated, non-tender, thyroid mass, possible lymphadenopathy.

Over-40s

Neck lumps are malignant until proven otherwise.
• Metastatic lymphadenopathy: multiple, rock hard, non-tender, tendency to be fixed.
• 75% in primary head and neck (thyroid, nasopharynx, tonsils, larynx, pharynx), 25% from infraclavicular primary (stomach, pancreas, lung).
• Primary lymphadenopathy (thyroid, lymphoma): fleshy, matted, rubbery, large size.
• Primary neoplasm (thyroid, salivary tumour): firm, non-tender, fixed to tissue of origin.

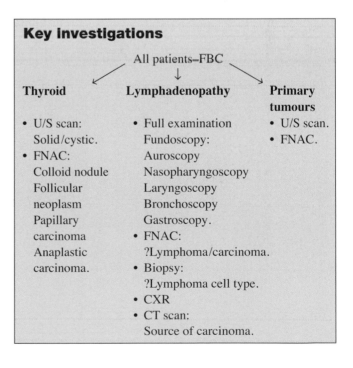

> ### Key Investigations
>
> All patients—FBC
>
> **Thyroid**
> • U/S scan: Solid/cystic.
> • FNAC: Colloid nodule Follicular neoplasm Papillary carcinoma Anaplastic carcinoma.
>
> **Lymphadenopathy**
> • Full examination Fundoscopy: Auroscopy Nasopharyngoscopy Laryngoscopy Bronchoscopy Gastroscopy.
> • FNAC: ?Lymphoma/carcinoma.
> • Biopsy: ?Lymphoma cell type.
> • CXR
> • CT scan: Source of carcinoma.
>
> **Primary tumours**
> • U/S scan.
> • FNAC.

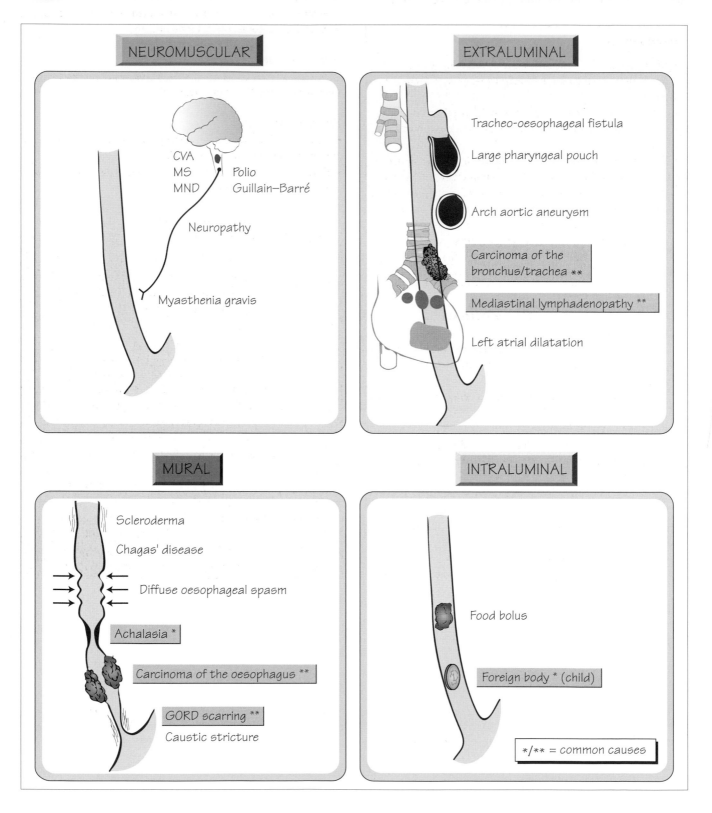

NEUROMUSCULAR

CVA
MS
MND

Polio
Guillain–Barré

Neuropathy

Myasthenia gravis

EXTRALUMINAL

Tracheo-oesophageal fistula

Large pharyngeal pouch

Arch aortic aneurysm

Carcinoma of the bronchus/trachea **

Mediastinal lymphadenopathy **

Left atrial dilatation

MURAL

Scleroderma

Chagas' disease

Diffuse oesophageal spasm

Achalasia *

Carcinoma of the oesophagus **

GORD scarring **

Caustic stricture

INTRALUMINAL

Food bolus

Foreign body * (child)

*/** = common causes

Definition

Dysphagia literally means difficulty with swallowing, which may be associated with ingestion of solids or liquids or both.

Important diagnostic features

Mural causes

- Carcinoma of the oesophagus: progressive course, associated weight loss and anorexia, low-grade anaemia, possible small haematemesis.
- Reflux oesophagitis and stricture: preceded by heartburn, progressive course, nocturnal regurgitation (24-hour oesophageal pH monitoring may be indicated).
- Achalasia: onset in young adulthood or old age, liquids disproportionately difficult to swallow, frequent regurgitation, recurrent chest infections, long history.
- Tracheo-oesophageal fistula: recurrent chest infections, coughing after drinking. Present in infants (congenital) or late adulthood (post trauma, deep X-ray therapy (DXT) or malignant).
- Chagas' disease (*Trypanosoma cruzi*): South American prevalence, associated with dysrhythmias and colonic dysmotility.

- Caustic stricture: examination shows corrosive ingestion, chronic dysphagia, onset may be months after ingestion of caustic agent.
- Scleroderma: slow onset, associated with skin changes, Raynaud's phenomenon and mild arthritis.

Intraluminal causes

Foreign body: acute onset, marked retrosternal discomfort, dysphagia even to saliva is characteristic.

Extramural causes

- Pulsion diverticulum (pharyngeal pouch): intermittent symptoms, unexpected regurgitation.
- External compression: mediastinal lymph nodes, left atrial hypertrophy, bronchial malignancy.

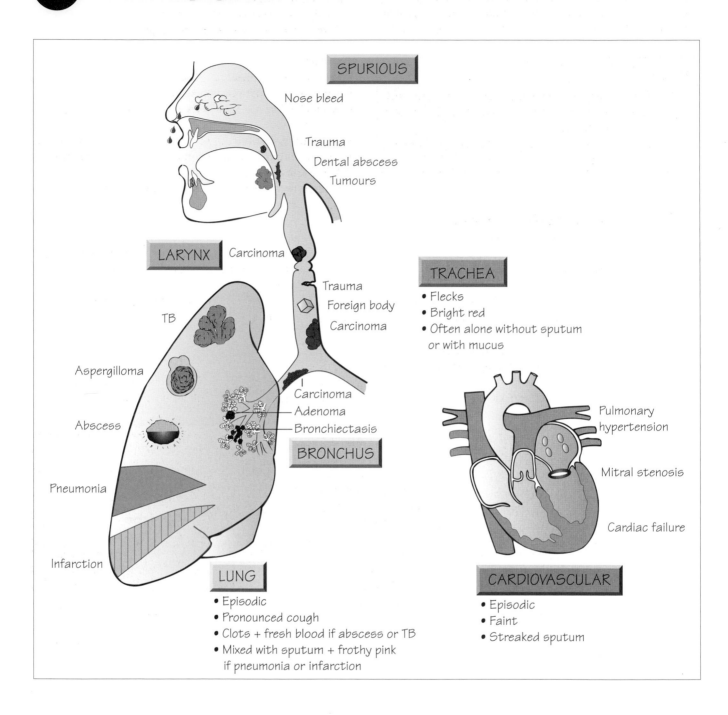

SPURIOUS

Nose bleed

Trauma

Dental abscess

Tumours

LARYNX

Carcinoma

TRACHEA
- Flecks
- Bright red
- Often alone without sputum or with mucus

Trauma

Foreign body

Carcinoma

TB

Aspergilloma

Carcinoma

Adenoma

Bronchiectasis

Abscess

BRONCHUS

Pneumonia

Infarction

LUNG
- Episodic
- Pronounced cough
- Clots + fresh blood if abscess or TB
- Mixed with sputum + frothy pink if pneumonia or infarction

Pulmonary hypertension

Mitral stenosis

Cardiac failure

CARDIOVASCULAR
- Episodic
- Faint
- Streaked sputum

Definition

Haemoptysis (blood spitting) is the symptom of coughing up blood from the lungs. Blood from the nose, mouth or pharynx that may also be spat out is termed 'spurious haemoptysis'.

Key points

- Blood from the proximal bronchi or trachea is usually bright red. It may be frankly blood or mixed with mucus and debris, particularly from a tumour.
- Blood from the distal bronchioles and alveoli is often pink and mixed with frothy sputum.

Important diagnostic features

The sources, causes and features are listed below.

Spurious haemoptysis
Mouth and nose

- Blood dyscrasias: associated nose bleeds, spontaneous bruising.
- Scurvy (vitamin C deficiency): poor hair/teeth, skin bruising.
- Dental caries, trauma, gingivitis.
- Oral tumours: painful intraoral mass, discharge, fetor.
- Hypertensive/spontaneous: no warning, brief bleed, often recurrent.
- Nasal tumours (common in South-East Asia).

True haemoptysis
Larynx and trachea

- Foreign body: choking, stridor, pain.
- Carcinoma: hoarse voice, bovine cough.

Bronchus

- Carcinoma: spontaneous haemoptysis, chest infections, weight loss, monophonic wheezing.
- Adenoma (e.g. carcinoid): recurrent chest infections, carcinoid syndrome.
- Bronchiectasis: chronic chest infections, fetor, blood mixed with copious purulent sputum; physical examination may show TB or severe chest infections.
- Foreign body: recurrent chest infections, sudden-onset inexplicable 'asthma'.

Lung

- TB: weight loss, fevers, night sweats, dry or productive cough.
- Pneumonia/lung abscess: features of acute chest sepsis, swinging fever.
- Pulmonary infarct (secondary to PE): pleuritic chest pain, tachypnoea, pleural rub.
- Aspergilloma.

Cardiac

- Mitral stenosis: frothy pink sputum, recurrent chest infections.
- LVF: frothy pink sputum, pulmonary oedema.

Key investigations

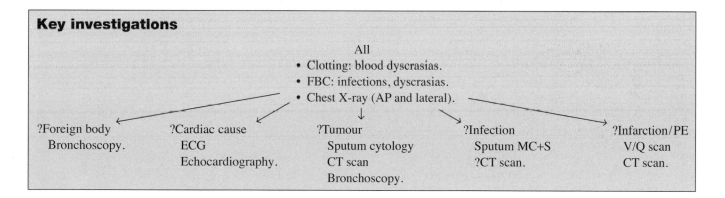

All
- Clotting: blood dyscrasias.
- FBC: infections, dyscrasias.
- Chest X-ray (AP and lateral).

?Foreign body	?Cardiac cause	?Tumour	?Infection	?Infarction/PE
Bronchoscopy.	ECG	Sputum cytology	Sputum MC+S	V/Q scan
	Echocardiography.	CT scan	?CT scan.	CT scan.
		Bronchoscopy.		

4 Breast lump

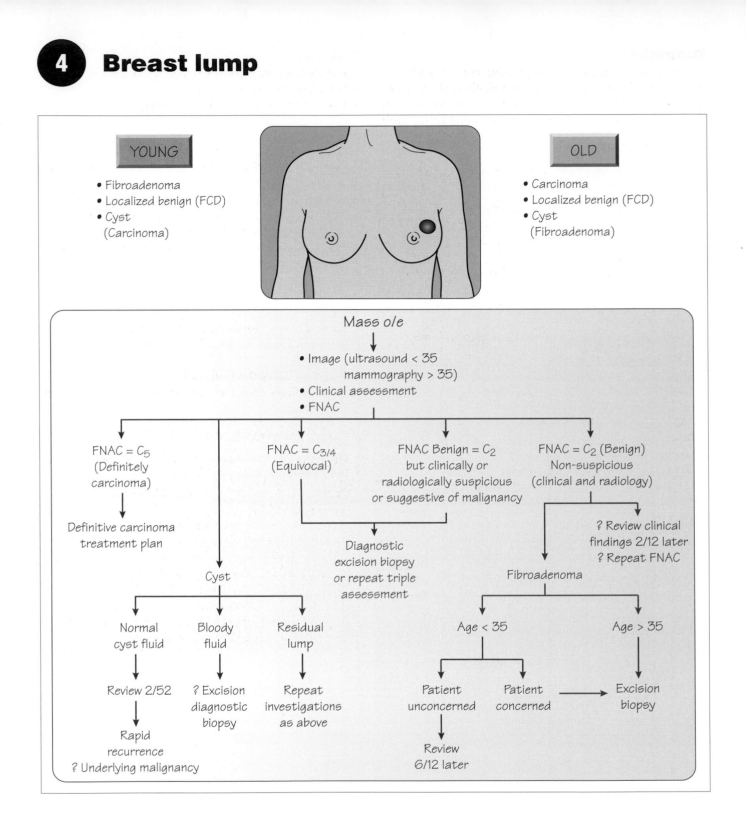

YOUNG
- Fibroadenoma
- Localized benign (FCD)
- Cyst
  (Carcinoma)

OLD
- Carcinoma
- Localized benign (FCD)
- Cyst
  (Fibroadenoma)

Mass o/e

- Image (ultrasound < 35
  mammography > 35)
- Clinical assessment
- FNAC

FNAC = C_5
(Definitely
carcinoma)

FNAC = $C_{3/4}$
(Equivocal)

FNAC Benign = C_2
but clinically or
radiologically suspicious
or suggestive of malignancy

FNAC = C_2 (Benign)
Non-suspicious
(clinical and radiology)

Definitive carcinoma
treatment plan

? Review clinical
findings 2/12 later
? Repeat FNAC

Diagnostic
excision biopsy
or repeat triple
assessment

Cyst

Fibroadenoma

Normal
cyst fluid

Bloody
fluid

Residual
lump

Age < 35

Age > 35

Review 2/52

? Excision
diagnostic
biopsy

Repeat
investigations
as above

Patient
unconcerned

Patient
concerned

Excision
biopsy

Rapid
recurrence
? Underlying malignancy

Review
6/12 later

Definition

A *breast lump* is defined as any palpable mass in the breast. A breast lump is the most common presentation of both benign and malignant breast disease. Enlargement of the whole breast can occur either uni- or bilaterally, but this is not strictly a breast lump.

Key points

- The most common breast lumps occurring under the age of 35 years are fibroadenomas and fibrocystic disease.
- The most common breast lumps occurring over the age of 50 years are carcinomas and cysts.
- Pain is more characteristic of infection/inflammation than tumours.
- Skin/chest wall tethering is more characteristic of tumours than benign disease.
- Multiple lesions are usually benign (cysts or fibrocystic disease).

Differential diagnosis

Swelling of the whole breast

Bilateral
- Pregnancy, lactation.
- Idiopathic hypertrophy.
- Drug induced (e.g. diethylstilbestrol, cimetidine).

Unilateral
- Enlargement in the newborn.
- Puberty.

Localized swellings in the breast

Mastitis/breast abscess
- During lactation: red, hot, tender lump, systemic upset.
- Tuberculous abscess: chronic, 'cold', recurrent, discharging sinus.

Cysts
- Galactocele: more common postpartum, tender but not inflamed, milky contents.
- Fibrocystic disease: irregular, ill defined, often tender.

Solid lumps
Benign include:
- Fibroadenoma: discrete, firm, well defined, regular, highly mobile.
- Fat necrosis: irregular, ill defined, hard, ?skin tethering.
- Lipoma: well defined, soft, non-tender, fairly mobile.
- Cystosarcoma phylloides: usually large tumour (5 cm), firm, mobile, well circumscribed, non-tender breast mass. (rare, 1% of breast tumours, 10% are malignant).

Malignant include:
- Carcinoma
  early: ill defined, hard, irregular, skin tethering
  late: spreading fixity, ulceration, fungation, '*peau d'orange*'.

Swellings behind the breast
- Rib deformities, chondroma, costochondritis (Tietze's disease).

Key investigations

All lumps should have triple assessment (examination, FNAC, radiology)
- FNAC: tumours, fibroadenoma, fibrocystic disease, fat necrosis, mastitis.
- Ultrasound (better in young women with denser breasts): fibroadenoma, cysts, tumours.
- Mammography (better in older women with less dense breasts): tumours, cysts, fibrocystic disease, fat necrosis.
- Biopsy ('Trucut'/core, rarely open surgical): usually provides definitive histology (may be radiologically guided if lump is small or impalpable, *e.g.* detected by mammography as part of breast screening programme).

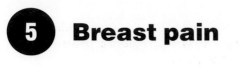

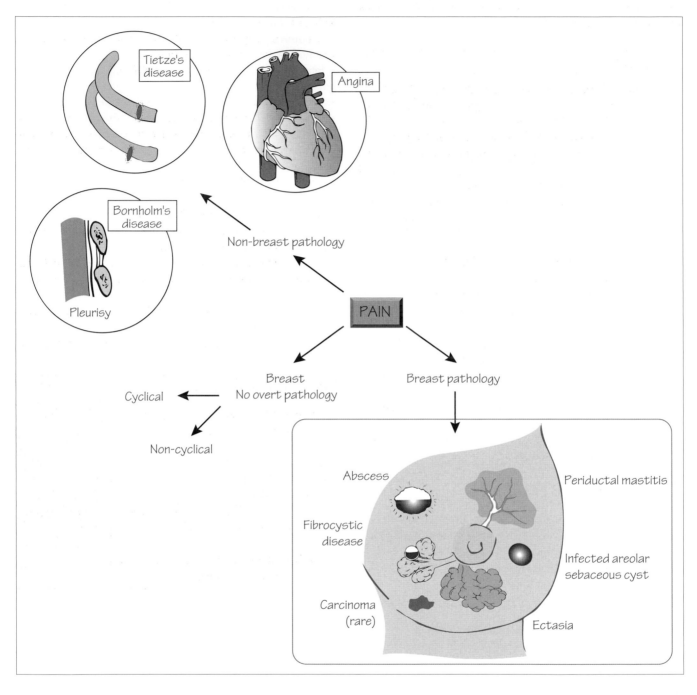

Tietze's disease

Angina

Bornholm's disease

Pleurisy

Non-breast pathology

PAIN

Breast
No overt pathology

Breast pathology

Cyclical

Non-cyclical

Abscess

Fibrocystic disease

Carcinoma (rare)

Periductal mastitis

Infected areolar sebaceous cyst

Ectasia

Definition

Mastalgia is any pain felt in the breast. *Cyclical mastalgia* is pain in the breast that varies in association with the menstrual cycle. *Non-cyclical mastalgia* is pain in the breast that follows no pattern or is intermittent.

Key points

• Mastalgia is commonly due to disorders of the breast or nipple tissue but may also be due to problems in the underlying chest wall or overlying skin.

• Pain is an uncommon presenting feature of tumours but any underlying lump should be investigated as for a lump (see Chapter 4).

• Always look for an associated infection in the breast.

• Mammography should be routine in women presenting over the age of 45 years to help exclude occult carcinoma.

Important diagnostic features

Non-breast conditions

• Tietze's disease (costochondritis): tenderness over medial ends of ribs, not limited to the breast area of the chest wall, relieved by NSAIDs.

• Bornholm's disease (epidemic pleurodynia caused by coxsackie A virus): marked pain with no physical signs in the breast, worse with inspiration, no chest disease underlying, relieved with NSAIDs.

• Pleurisy: associated chest infection, pleural rub, may be bilateral.

• Angina: usually atypical angina, may be hard to diagnose, previous history of associated vascular disease.

Mastalgia due to breast pathology

Mastitis/breast abscess

• During lactation: red hot tender lump, systemic upset:
   treatment: aspirate abscess (may need to be repeated), do not stop breastfeeding, oral antibiotics.

• Non-lactational abscesses: recurrent, associated with smoking, associated with underlying ductal ectasia:

treatment: outpatient aspiration, give oral antibiotics, stop smoking, prophylactic metronidazole for recurrent sepsis, repeat aspiration if necessary.

Infected sebaceous cyst

• Single lump superficially in the skin of the periareolar region, previous history of painless cystic lump:
   treatment: excise infected cyst ± antibiotics.

Fibrocystic disease

• Common condition. Breast discomfort, dull heavy pain and tenderness. Variable symptoms and intensity, worse premenstrually. Cobblestone consistency to breast on palpation—upper outer quadrants:
   • treatment: as for mastalgia.

Mastalgia without breast pathology

• Pain often felt throughout the breast, often worse in the axillary tail, moderately tender to examination:
   general treatment: restrict dietary fat and avoid caffeine, possibly vitamin E, well-fitting bra to provide good breast support
   treatment for cyclical mastalgia: γ linoleic acid (evening primrose oil), danazol, tamoxifen
   treatment for non-cyclical mastalgia: NSAIDs, γ linoleic acid.

Key investigations

Non-breast origin

Chest X-ray, ECG (exercise).

Breast pathology

• FNAC (MC+S): associated palpable lump, ?fibrocystic disease, ?mastitis/abscess.

• Ultrasound (young women/dense breasts) or mammography (older women/small breasts).

Mastalgia without breast pathology

Mammography in women over 45 years.

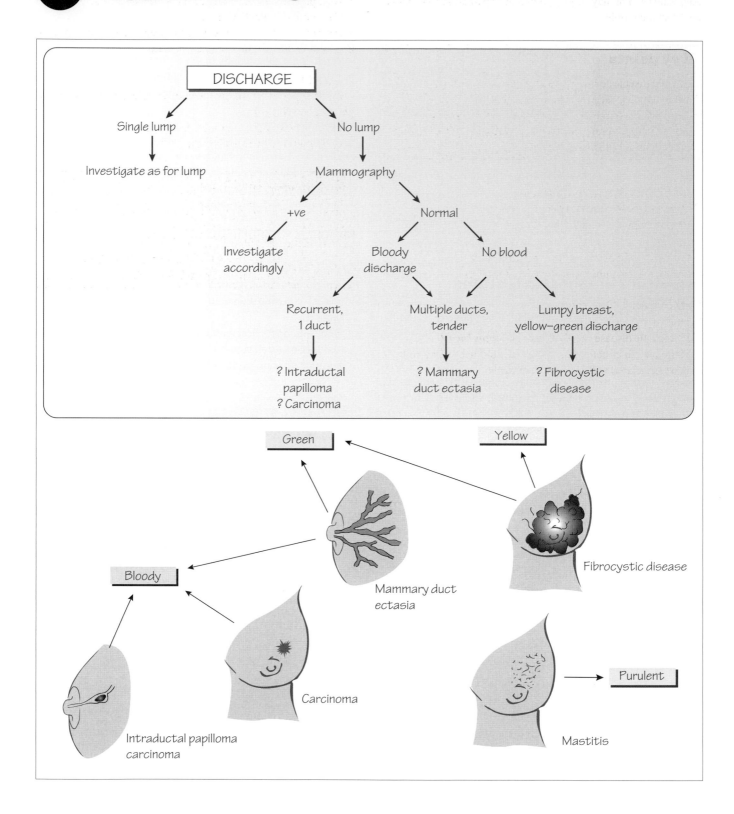

DISCHARGE

Single lump → Investigate as for lump

No lump → Mammography

+ve → Investigate accordingly

Normal → Bloody discharge / No blood

Recurrent, 1 duct → ? Intraductal papilloma ? Carcinoma

Multiple ducts, tender → ? Mammary duct ectasia

Lumpy breast, yellow–green discharge → ? Fibrocystic disease

Green

Yellow

Bloody

Mammary duct ectasia

Fibrocystic disease

Carcinoma

Intraductal papilloma carcinoma

Purulent

Mastitis

Definition

Any fluid (which may be physiological or pathological) emanating from the nipple.

Key points

- Milky discharge is rarely pathological.
- Purulent discharge is usually benign.
- Bloody discharge is often associated with neoplasia.
- If a lump is present, always investigate 'for the lump' rather than 'for the discharge'.

Differential diagnosis

Physiological discharges

Milky or clear

- Lactation.
- Lactorrhoea in the newborn ('witches' milk').
- Lactorrhoea at puberty (may be in either sex).

Pathological discharges

Serous yellow–green

- Fibrocystic disease: cyclical, tender, lumpy breasts.
- Mammary duct ectasia: usually multiple ducts, intermittent, may be associated with low-grade mastitis.

Bloody

- Duct papilloma: single duct, ?retro-areolar, 'pea-sized' lump.
- Carcinoma: ?palpable lump.
- Mammary duct ectasia: usually multiple ducts, intermittent, may be associated with low-grade mastitis.

Pus ± milk

- Acute suppurative mastitis: tender, swollen, hot breast, multiple ducts discharging.
- Tuberculous (rare): chronic discharge, periareolar fistulae, 'sterile' cultures on normal media.

Key investigations

- MC+S: acute mastitis, TB (Lowenstein–Jensen medium, Ziehl–Neelsen stains).
- Discharge cytology: carcinoma.
- Mammography: tumours, fibrocystic disease, ?ectasla.
- Ductal excision: may be needed for exclusion of neoplasia.

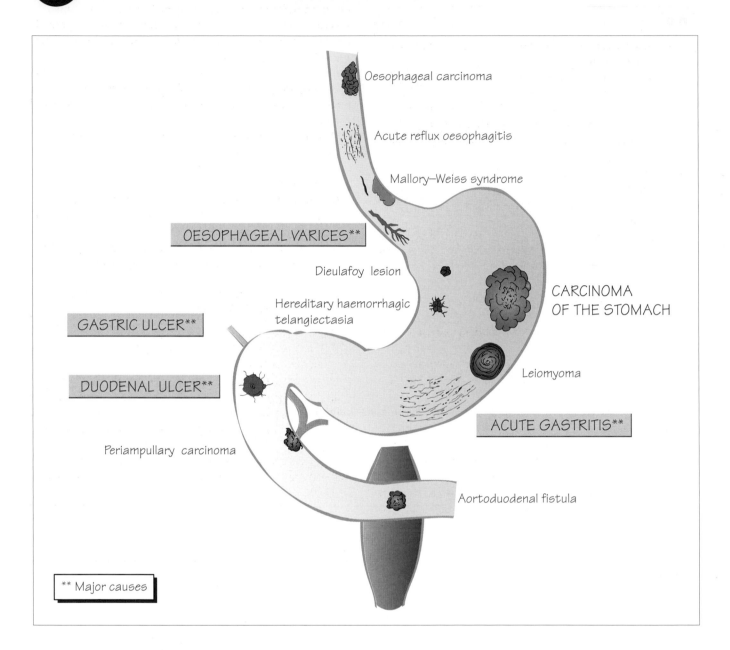

Oesophageal carcinoma

Acute reflux oesophagitis

Mallory–Weiss syndrome

OESOPHAGEAL VARICES**

Dieulafoy lesion

Hereditary haemorrhagic telangiectasia

GASTRIC ULCER**

DUODENAL ULCER**

Periampullary carcinoma

CARCINOMA OF THE STOMACH

Leiomyoma

ACUTE GASTRITIS**

Aortoduodenal fistula

** Major causes

Definitions

GI bleeding is any blood loss from the GI tract (anywhere from the mouth to the anus), which may present with haematemesis, melaena, rectal bleeding or anaemia. *Haematemesis* is defined as vomiting blood and is usually caused by upper GI disease.

Melaena is the passage PR of a black treacle-like stool that contains altered blood, usually as a result of proximal bowel bleeding. *Haematochesia* is the presence of undigested blood in the stool usually from lower GI causes.

Upper GI bleeding

Key points

- Haematemesis is usually caused by lesions proximal to the duodeno-jejunal junction.
- Melaena may be caused by lesions anywhere from oesophagus to colon.
- Haematochesia is usually caused by lower GI pathology (colorectal tumours, haemorrhoids, diverticulitis, angiodysplasia) although brisk acute small intestinal bleeding may present this way.
- Most tumours more commonly cause anaemia than frank haematemesis.
- In young adults, PUD, congenital lesions and varices are common causes.
- In the elderly, tumours, PUD and angiodysplasia are common causes.

Important diagnostic features
Oesophagus

- Reflux oesophagitis: small volumes, bright red, associated with regurgitation.
- Oesophageal carcinoma (rare): scanty, bloodstained debris, rarely significant volume, associated with weight loss, anergia, dysphagia.
- Bleeding varices (oesophageal or gastric): sudden onset, painless, large volumes, dark red blood, history of (alcoholic) liver disease, other features of portal hypertension (ascites, dilated abdominal veins, encephalopathy, reduced platelets or white cells).
- Trauma during vomiting (Mallory–Weiss syndrome): bright red bloody vomit usually preceded by several normal but forceful vomiting episodes.

Stomach

- Erosive gastritis: small volumes, bright red, may follow alcohol or NSAID intake/stress, history of dyspeptic symptoms.
- Gastric ulcer: often larger sized bleed, painless, possible herald smaller bleeds, accompanied by altered blood ('coffee grounds'), history of PUD.
- Gastric cancer: rarely large bleed, anaemia more common, associated weight loss, anorexia, dyspeptic symptoms.
- Gastric leiomyoma (rare): spontaneous-onset moderate-sized bleed.
- Dieulafoy's disease (rare): younger patients, spontaneous large bleed, difficult to diagnose.

Duodenum

- Duodenal ulcer: past history of duodenal ulcer, melaena often also prominent, symptoms of back pain, hunger pains, NSAID use.
- Aorto-duodenal fistula (rare): usually infected graft post AAA repair, massive haematemesis and PR bleed, usually fatal.

Key investigations

- FBC: carcinomas, reflux oesophagitis.
- LFTs: liver disease (varices).
- Clotting: alcohol, bleeding diatheses.
- OGD: investigation of choice. High diagnostic accuracy, allows therapeutic manoeuvres also (varices: injection; ulcers: injection/cautery).
- Angiography: rare duodenal causes, obscure recurrent bleeds.
- Barium meal and follow through: useful for patients who are unfit for OGD (respiratory disease) and ?proximal jejunal lesions.

Essential management

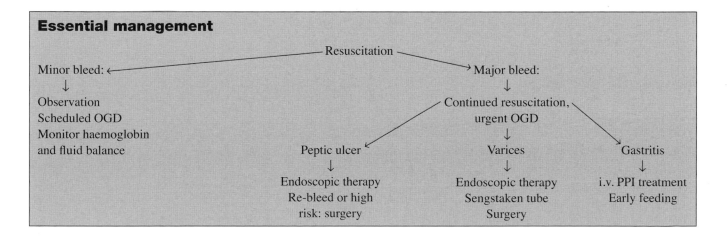

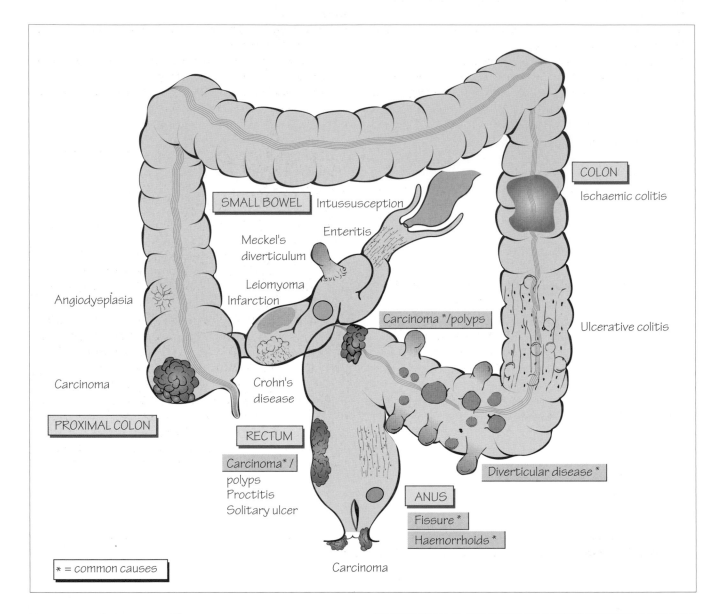

In the figure the following labels appear:

SMALL BOWEL Intussusception

COLON

Ischaemic colitis

Enteritis

Meckel's diverticulum

Leiomyoma
Infarction

Angiodysplasia

Carcinoma */polyps

Ulcerative colitis

Carcinoma

Crohn's disease

PROXIMAL COLON

RECTUM

Carcinoma*/
polyps
Proctitis
Solitary ulcer

Diverticular disease *

ANUS

Fissure *

Haemorrhoids *

* = common causes

Carcinoma

Lower GI bleeding

Key points

• Anorectal bleeding is characteristically bright red, associated with defaecation, not mixed with the stool and visible on toilet paper—often associated with other symptoms of anorectal disease.

• Distal (left-sided/sigmoid) bleeding is characteristically dark red, with clots, may be mixed with the stool.

• Proximal colonic or ileal bleeding is characteristically dark red, fully mixed with the stool or occult—unless heavy when it may appear as 'distal' or 'anorectal' in type.

• In children, acute anal fissure, Meckel's diverticulum, intussusception and ileal tumours are common causes.

• In young adults, colitis, Meckel's diverticulum, anal fissure and haemorrhoids are common causes.

• In the elderly, neoplasia, diverticular disease and angiodysplasia are common causes.

• Always perform a rectal examination and rigid sigmoidoscopy in all patients.

• New rectal bleeding age >55 always deserves colonic investigation—never assume it is a simple anal cause.

• Bright red bleeding with no obvious anal cause requires at least a flexible sigmoidoscopy.

• Any suggestion of dark red blood or a +ve FOB requires colonic imaging or colonoscopy.

• Acute major PR bleeding is usually due to diverticular disease, angiodysplsia, Meckel's diverticulum related ulceration or haemorrhoids.

Important diagnostic features

Small intestine

- Meckel's diverticulum: young adults, painless bleeding, darker red/melaena common.
- Intussusception: young children, colicky abdominal pain, retching, bright red/mucus stool.
- Enteritis (infective/radiation/Crohn's disease).
- Ischaemic: severe abdominal pain, physical examination shows mesenteric ischaemia or AF, few signs, later collapse and shock.
- Tumours (leiomyoma/lymphoma): rare, intermittent history, often modest volumes lost.

Proximal colon

- Angiodysplasia: common in the elderly, painless, no warning, often large volume, fresh and clots mixed.
- Carcinoma of the caecum: more often causes anaemia than PR bleeding.

Colon

- Polyps/carcinoma: may be large volume or small, ?associated change in bowel habit, blood often mixed with stool.
- Diverticular disease: spontaneous onset, painless, large volume, mostly fresh blood, previous history of constipation.
- Ulcerative colitis: blood mixed with mucus, associated with systemic upset, long history, intermittent course, diarrhoea prominent.
- Ischaemic colitis: elderly, severe abdominal pain, AF, bloody diarrhoea, collapse and shock later.

Rectum

- Carcinoma of the rectum: change in bowel habit common, rarely large volumes.
- Proctitis: bloody mucus, purulent diarrhoea in infected, perianal irritation common.
- Solitary rectal ulcer: bleeding post defaecation, small volumes, feeling of 'lump in anus', mucus discharge.

Anus

- Haemorrhoids: bright red bleeding post defaecation, stops spontaneously, perianal irritation.
- Fissure *in ano*: extreme pain post defaecation, small volumes bright red blood on stool and toilet paper.
- Carcinoma of the anus: elderly, mass in anus, small volumes bloody discharge, anal pain, unhealing ulcers.
- Perianal Crohn's disease.

Key investigations

- FBC: anaemia—tumours/chronic colitis.
- Clotting: bleeding diatheses.
- PR/sigmoidoscopy: anorectal tumours, prolapse, haemorrhoids, distal colitis.
- Abdominal X-ray: intussusception.
- Flexible sigmoidoscopy: suspected anorectal cause.
- Colonoscopy: diverticular disease, colitis, colonic tumours, angiodysplasia.
- Angiography (CT or conventional): angiodysplasia, small bowel causes (especially Meckel's diverticulum). (Needs active bleeding 0.5 mL/min, highly accurate when positive, invasive, conventional allows embolization therapy.)
- Technetium-99m-pertechnate labelled RBC scan: angiodysplasia, small bowel causes including Meckel's diverticulum, obscure colonic causes. (Needs active bleeding 1 mL/min, less accurate placement of source, non-invasive, non-therapeutic.)
- Small bowel enema: small bowel tumours/angiodyplasia.

Essential management of acute IGI bleeding

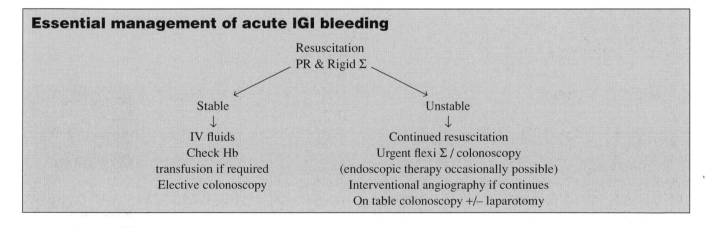

8 Dyspepsia

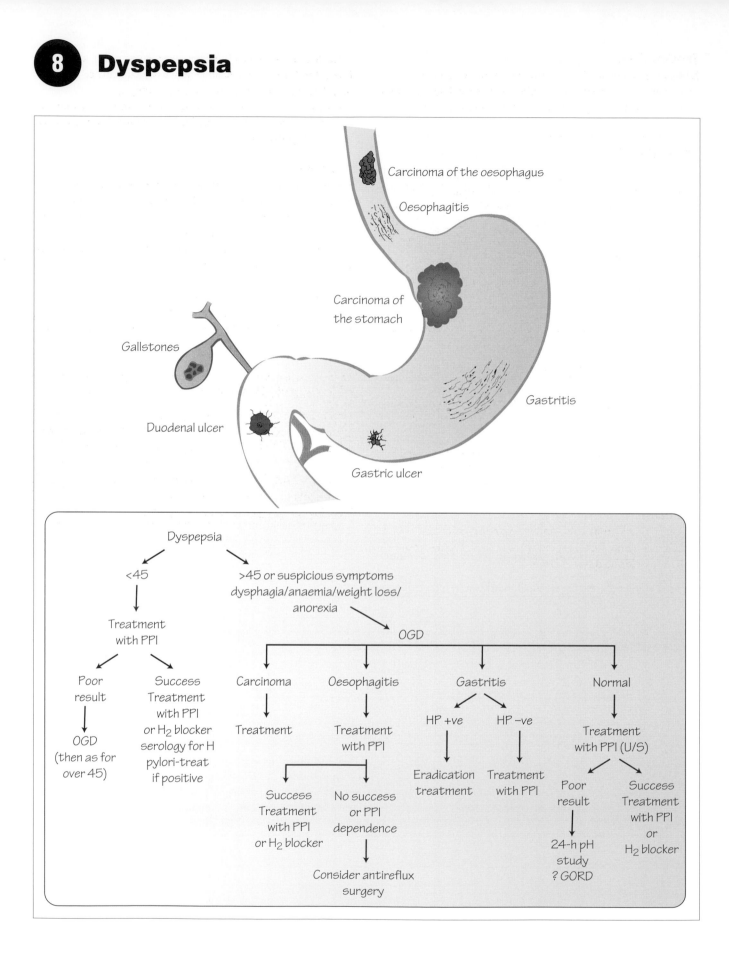

Definition

Dyspepsia is the feeling of discomfort or pain in the upper abdomen or lower chest. *Indigestion* may be used by the patient to mean dyspepsia, regurgitation symptoms or flatulence.

> ## Key points
>
> • Dyspepsia may be the only presenting symptom of upper GI malignancy. All older patients and patients with alarm symptoms (dysphagia, vomiting, anorexia and weight loss, GI bleeding) should have endoscopy.
> • Dyspepsia in young people without alarm symptoms is very unlikely to be due to malignancy.
> • In young adults, gastro-oesophageal reflux and *Helicobacter pylori*-positive gastritis are common causes.
> • Dyspepsia is rarely the only symptom of gallstones—they are more often incidental findings.

Differential diagnosis

Oesophagus

• Reflux oesophagitis: retrosternal dyspepsia, worse after large meal/lying down, associated symptoms of regurgitation, pain on swallowing.
• Oesophageal carcinoma: new-onset dyspepsia in older patient, associated symptoms of dysphagia/weight loss/haematemesis, failure to respond to acid suppression treatment.

Stomach

• Gastritis: recurrent episodes of epigastric pain, transient or short-lived symptoms, may be associated with diet, responds well to antacids/acid suppression.
• Gastric ulcer: typically chronic epigastric pain, worse with food, 'food fear' may lead to weight loss, exacerbated by smoking/alcohol, occasionally relieved by vomiting.
• Carcinoma of the stomach: progressive symptoms, associated weight loss/anorexia, iron-deficient anaemia common, early satiety, epigastric mass.

Duodenum

• Duodenal ulcer: epigastric and back pain, chronic exacerbations lasting several weeks, relieved by food especially milky drinks, relieved by bed rest, more common in younger men, associated with *H. pylori* infection.
• Duodenitis: often transient, mild symptoms only, associated with alcohol and smoking.

Gallstones

Dyspepsia is rarely the only symptom, associated RUQ pain, needs normal OGD and positive ultrasound to be considered as cause for dyspeptic symptoms.

> ## Key investigations
>
> • FBC: anaemia suggests malignancy.
> • Tests for *H. pylori*: breath test (C14 or C13 urea), blood (antibodies to *H. pylori*) or endoscopic biopsy urease test (CLO test).
> • OGD: tumours, PUD, assessment of oesophagitis.
> • 24-hour pH monitoring: ?GORD.
> • Ultrasound: ?gallstones.

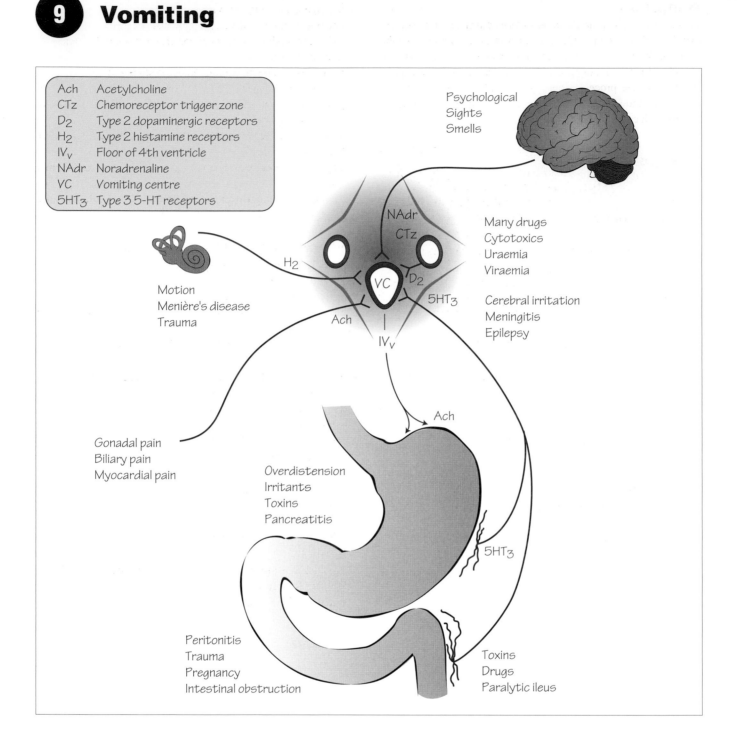

Ach   Acetylcholine
CTz   Chemoreceptor trigger zone
D_2 Type 2 dopaminergic receptors
H_2 Type 2 histamine receptors
IV_v Floor of 4th ventricle
NAdr   Noradrenaline
VC   Vomiting centre
$5HT_3$ Type 3 5-HT receptors

Psychological
Sights
Smells

NAdr
CTz
H_2
VC
D_2
$5HT_3$
Ach
IV_v

Many drugs
Cytotoxics
Uraemia
Viraemia

Cerebral irritation
Meningitis
Epilepsy

Motion
Menière's disease
Trauma

Ach

Gonadal pain
Biliary pain
Myocardial pain

Overdistension
Irritants
Toxins
Pancreatitis

$5HT_3$

Peritonitis
Trauma
Pregnancy
Intestinal obstruction

Toxins
Drugs
Paralytic ileus

Definitions

Vomiting is defined as the involuntary return to, and forceful expulsion from, the mouth of all or part of the contents of the stomach. *Waterbrash* is the sudden secretion and accumulation of saliva in the mouth as a reflex associated with dyspepsia. *Retching* is the process whereby forceful contractions of the diaphragm and abdominal muscles occur without evacuation of the stomach contents.

Key points

• Vomiting is initiated when the vomiting centre in the medulla oblongata is stimulated, either directly (central vomiting) or via various afferent fibres (reflex vomiting).
• Vomiting of different origins is mediated by different pathways and transmitters. Therapy is best directed according to cause.
• Consider mechanical causes (e.g. gastric outflow or intestinal obstruction) before starting therapy.

Important diagnostic features

Central vomiting

• Drugs, e.g. morphine sulphate, chemotherapeutic agents.
• Uraemia.
• Viral hepatitis.
• Hypercalcaemia of any cause.
• Acute infections, especially in children.
• Pregnancy.

Reflex vomiting

Gastrointestinal causes (5-HT$_3$ and Ach mediated—treatment: promotilants, 5-HT$_3$ antagonists)

• Ingestion of irritants:
  bacteria, e.g. salmonella (gastroenteritis)
  emetics, e.g. zinc sulphate, ipecacuanha
  drugs, e.g. alcohol, salicylates (gastritis)
  poisons, e.g. salt, arsenic, phosphorus.
• PUD: especially gastric ulcer; vomiting relieves the pain.
• Intestinal obstruction:
  hour-glass stomach (carcinoma of the stomach)
  pyloric stenosis—infant: hypertrophic pyloric stenosis, projectile vomiting; adult: pyloric outlet obstruction secondary to PUD or malignant disease
  small bowel obstruction: adhesions, hernia, neoplasm, Crohn's disease
  large bowel obstruction: malignancy, volvulus, diverticular disease.
• Inflammation: appendicitis, peritonitis, pancreatitis, cholecystitis, biliary colic.

General causes (Ach and D$_2$ mediated—treatment: anticholinergics, antidopaminergics)

• Myocardial infarction.
• Ovarian disease, ectopic pregnancy.
• Severe pain (e.g. kick to the testis, gonadal torsion, blow to the epigastrium).
• Severe coughing (e.g. pulmonary TB, pertussis).

CNS causes (NAdr and Ach mediated—treatment: anticholinergics, sedatives)

• Raised intracranial pressure:
  head injury
  cerebral tumour or abscess
  hydrocephalus
  meningitis
  cerebral haemorrhage.
• Migraine.
• Epilepsy.
• Offensive sights, tastes and smells.
• Hysteria.
• Middle ear disorders (H$_2$ mediated—treatment: antihistamines):
  Menière's disease
  travel/motion sickness

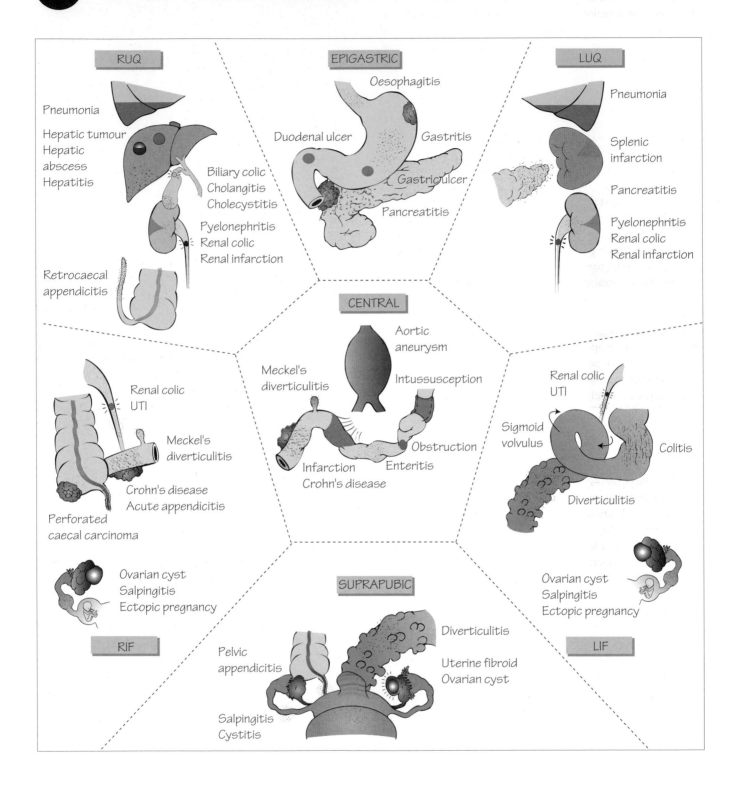

Definitions

Abdominal pain is a subjective unpleasant sensation felt in any of the abdominal regions. *Acute abdominal pain* is usually used to refer to pain of sudden onset, and/or short duration. *Referred pain* is the perception of pain in an area remote from the site of origin of the pain.

Key points

• The site of abdominal pain generally relates to its origin: foregut—upper; midgut—middle; hindgut—lower.
• Generally, colicky (visceral) pain is caused by stretching or contracting a hollow viscus (e.g. gallbladder, ureter, ileum).
• Generally, constant localized (somatic) pain is caused by peritoneal irritation and indicates the presence of inflammation/infection (e.g. pancreatitis, cholecystitis, appendicitis).
• Associated back pain suggests retroperitoneal pathology (aortic aneurysm, pancreatitis, posterior DU, pyelonephritis).
• Associated sacral or perineal pain suggests pelvic pathology (ovarian cyst, PID, pelvic abscess).
• Generally, very severe pain indicates ischaemia or generalized peritonitis (e.g. mesenteric infarction, perforated DU).
• Pain out of proportion to the physical signs suggests ischaemia without perforation.
• Remember referred causes of pain: pneumonia (right lower lobe), myocardial infarction, lumbar nerve root pathology.

Key investigations

FBC: leucocytosis—infective/inflammatory diseases; anaemia—occult malignancy, PUD.
• LFTs: usually abnormal in cholangitis, may be abnormal in acute cholecystitis.
• Amylase: serum level >3× upper limit of normal range is diagnostic of pancreatitis. Serum level 2–3× upper limit of normal range—?pancreatitis, perforated ulcer, bowel ischaemia, severe sepsis. Serum level raised mildly (up to 2×) non-specific indicator of pathology.
• β-HCG (serum): ectopic pregnancy (serum level is more accurate than urinary hormone).
• Arterial blood gases: metabolic acidosis—?bowel ischaemia, peritonitis, pancreatitis.
• MSU: urinary tract infection (++ve nitrites, blood, protein), renal stone (++ve blood).

• ECG: myocardial infarction.
• Chest X-ray: perforated viscus (free gas), pneumonia.
• Abdominal X-ray:
 ischaemic bowel (dilated, thickened oedematous loops)
 pancreatitis ('sentinel' dilated upper jejunum)
 cholangitis (air in biliary tree)
 acute colitis (dilated, oedematous, featureless colon)
 acute obstruction (dilated loops, 'string of pearls' sign)
 renal stones (radiodense opacity in renal tract).
• Ultrasound:
 intra-abdominal abscesses (diverticular, appendicular, pelvic)
 acute cholecystitis/empyema
 ovarian pathology (cyst, ectopic pregnancy)
 trauma (liver/spleen haematoma)
 renal infections.
• OGD: PUD, gastritis.
• CT scan: the investigation of choice for:
 undiagnosed peritoneal inflammation (particularly in the elderly where the differential diagnosis is wide
 patients for whom laparotomy is considered and the diagnosis is uncertain
 possible pancreatitis, trauma (liver/spleen/mesenteric injuries), diverticulitis, leaking aortic aneurysm.
• IVU: renal stones, renal tract obstruction.
• Diagnostic laparoscopy: possible appendicitis, tubo-ovarian disease, other causes of peritonitis—may be used for treatment.

Essential management

• Establish IV access and give fluids as necessary.
• Catheterize if hypotensive on presentation.
• Give opiate analgesia as required—it never masks true physical signs.
• Do not give IV antibiotics unless the diagnosis has been made or definitive investigations are planned (e.g. CT scan or laparoscopy).
• Observational management ('masterful inactivity') may be used for 24 hours in stable patients without signs of significant peritoneal inflammation.
• Investigate as appropriate.
• Consider laparosocopy especially in younger patients where symptoms or signs persist but the diagnosis remains unclear.

11 **Chronic abdominal pain**

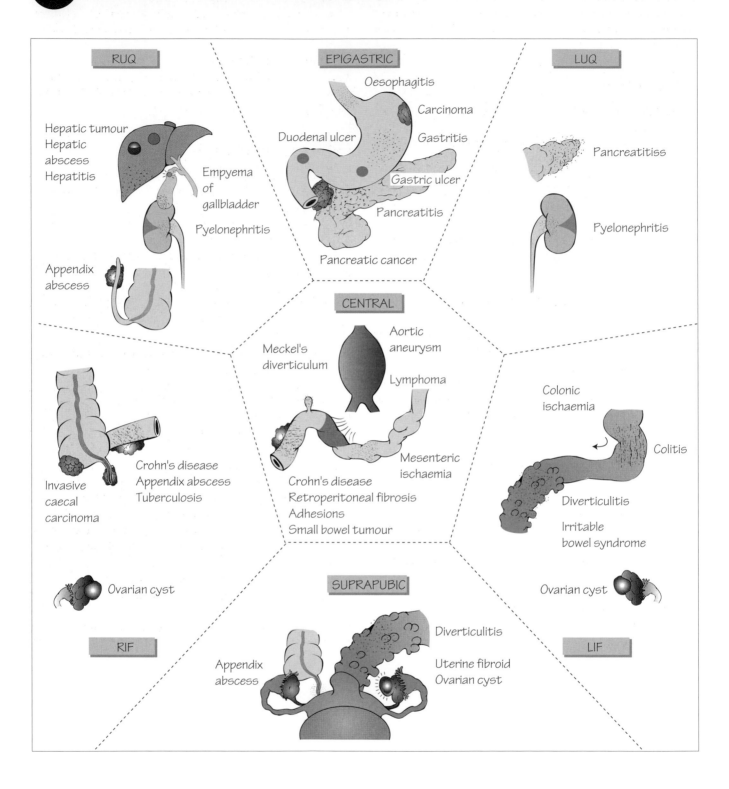

RUQ

Hepatic tumour
Hepatic abscess
Hepatitis

Empyema of gallbladder

Pyelonephritis

Appendix abscess

EPIGASTRIC

Oesophagitis

Carcinoma

Duodenal ulcer

Gastritis

Gastric ulcer

Pancreatitis

Pancreatic cancer

LUQ

Pancreatitiss

Pyelonephritis

CENTRAL

Meckel's diverticulum

Aortic aneurysm

Lymphoma

Mesenteric ischaemia

Crohn's disease
Retroperitoneal fibrosis
Adhesions
Small bowel tumour

Crohn's disease
Appendix abscess
Tuberculosis

Invasive caecal carcinoma

Colonic ischaemia

Colitis

Diverticulitis

Irritable bowel syndrome

Ovarian cyst

Ovarian cyst

RIF

SUPRAPUBIC

Appendix abscess

Diverticulitis

Uterine fibroid
Ovarian cyst

LIF

Definition

Chronic abdominal pain is usually used to refer to pain that is either long-standing, of prolonged duration or of recurrent/intermittent nature. Chronic pain may be associated with acute exacerbations.

Key points

- Chronic abdominal pain of prolonged duration requires investigation.
- Adhesions as a cause of chronic abdominal pain should be a diagnosis of exclusion.
- IBS is less common than supposed—any atypical bowel symptoms should be investigated fully before diagnosing IBS.
- Back pain suggests a retroperitoneal origin.
- Sacral pain suggests a pelvic origin.
- Relationship to food strongly suggests a physical pathology and requires investigation.

Important diagnostic features

Irritable bowel syndrome

- Syndrome of colicky abdominal pain, bloating, hard pellety or watery stools, sensation of incomplete evacuation, often associated with frequency and urgency.
- Blood, mucus, abdominal physical findings, weight loss or recent onset of symptoms or onset in old age should suggest an organic cause and require thorough investigation.

Adhesions

Associated with several syndromes of chronic or recurrent abdominal symptoms.

Adhesional abdominal pain

Difficult to diagnosis with any confidence, usually a diagnosis of exclusion, may be suggested by small bowel enema showing evidence of delayed transit or fixed strictures, rarely responds well to surgery.

Recurrent incomplete small bowel obstruction

Transient episodes of obstructive symptoms, often do not have all classic signs or symptoms present, abdominal signs may be unremarkable, self-limiting.

Mesenteric angina

Classically occurs shortly after eating in elderly patients, colicky central abdominal pain, vomiting, food fear and weight loss. Usually associated with other occlusive vascular disease.

Meckel's diverticulum

May cause undiagnosed central abdominal pain in young adults. Occasionally associated with obscure PR bleeding, anaemia. Best diagnosed by radionuclide scanning.

Key investigations

- FBC: leucocytosis—chronic infective/inflammatory diseases, anaemia—occult malignancy, PUD, lymphocytosis—lymphoma.
- LFTs: common bile duct gallstones, hepatitis, liver tumours (primary/secondary).
- MSU: urinary tract infection (++ve nitrites, blood, protein), renal stone (++ve blood).
- ECG: ischaemic heart disease.
- Abdominal X-ray: chronic pancreatitis (small calcification throughout gland):
- Ultrasound:
  intra-abdominal abscesses (diverticular, appendicular, pelvic, hepatic)
  'gallstones', 'chronic cholecystitis'
  ovarian pathology (cyst)
  aortic aneurysm, renal tumours
- OGD: PUD, gastritis, gastric or oesophageal carcinoma.
- Colonoscopy: diverticular disease, chronic colonic ischaemia, colonic polyps and tumours.
- CT scan: chronic pancreatitis, pancreatic carcinoma, aortic aneurysm, retroperitoneal pathologies (fibrosis, lymphadenopathy, tumours), bowel tumours.
- IVU: renal stones, renal tract tumours, renal tract obstruction.
- Visceral angiography/CT angiogram/mesenteric MRA: mesenteric vascular disease.
- ERCP: chronic pancreatitis, pancreatic carcinoma.
- Small bowel enema: Crohn's disease, small bowel tumours, Meckel's diverticulum.
- Barium enema: ischaemic strictures, chronic colitis.

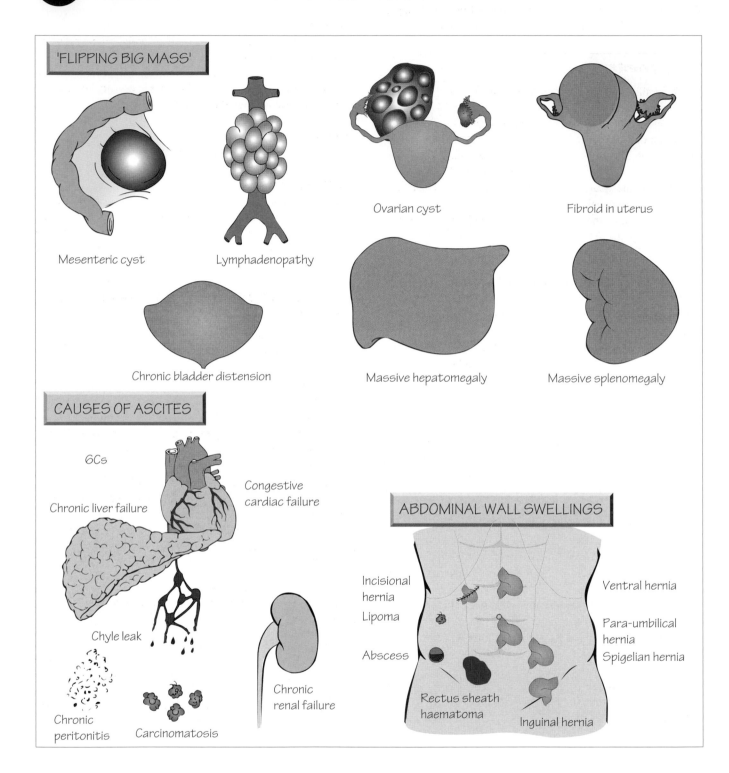

'FLIPPING BIG MASS'

Mesenteric cyst

Lymphadenopathy

Ovarian cyst

Fibroid in uterus

Chronic bladder distension

Massive hepatomegaly

Massive splenomegaly

CAUSES OF ASCITES

6Cs

Chronic liver failure

Congestive cardiac failure

Chyle leak

Chronic peritonitis

Carcinomatosis

Chronic renal failure

ABDOMINAL WALL SWELLINGS

Incisional hernia

Lipoma

Abscess

Rectus sheath haematoma

Inguinal hernia

Ventral hernia

Para-umbilical hernia

Spigelian hernia

Definition

An abdominal swelling is an abnormal protuberance that arises from the abdominal cavity or the abdominal wall and may be general or localized, acute or chronic, cystic or solid.

Key points

- Generalized abdominal swellings affect the entire abdominal cavity.
- Localized swellings can be located in the various regions of the abdomen.
- Abdominal wall swellings can be differentiated from intra-abdominal swellings by asking the patient to raise his or her head from the couch (intraperitoneal swellings disappear while abdominal wall swellings persist).
- Giant masses, other than ovarian cystadenocarcinoma, are rarely malignant.

Important diagnostic features

'Fat'

Obesity: deposition of fat in the abdominal wall and intra-abdominally (extraperitoneal layer, omentum and mesentery). Clinical obesity is present when a person's body weight is 120% greater than that recommended for their height, age and sex (BMI = weight (kg)/height (m)^2. A BMI of >25 is overweight, >30 obese.

'Flatus'

Intestinal obstruction: swallowed air accumulates in the bowel causing distension. This gives a tympanic note on percussion and produces the characteristic air–fluid levels and 'ladder' pattern on an abdominal radiograph. Sigmoid or caecal volvulus produces gross distension with characteristic features of distended loops on abdominal X-ray.

'Fluid'

- Intestinal obstruction: as well as air, fluid accumulates in the obstructed intestine.
- Ascites: fluid accumulates in the peritoneal cavity due to the '6 Cs':
  chronic peritonitis (e.g. tuberculosis, missed appendicitis)
  carcinomatosis (malignant deposits, especially ovary, stomach)
  chronic liver disease (cirrhosis, secondary deposits, portal or hepatic vein obstruction, parasitic infections)
  congestive heart failure (RVF)
  chronic renal failure (nephrotic syndrome)
  chyle (lymphatic duct disruption).

'Faeces'

Chronic constipation: faeces accumulate in the colon producing abdominal distension. Congenital causes include spina bifida and Hirschsprung's disease. Acquired causes include emotional disorders, chronic dehydration, drugs (opiates, anticholinergics, phenothiazines) and hypothyroidism.

'Fetus'

Pregnancy: swelling arises out of the pelvis.

'Flipping big mass'

Usually cystic lesions: giant ovarian cystadenoma, mesenteric cyst, retroperitoneal lymphadenopathy (lymphoma), giant uterine fibroid, giant splenomegaly, giant hepatomegaly, giant renal tumour, desmoid tumour. Occasionally, very distended bladder.

Key investigations—*abdominal masses*

- FBC: lymphomas, infections.
- LFT: liver disease.
- U+E: renal disease.
- Abdominal X-ray:
  ascites ('ground glass' appearance, loss of visceral outlines)
  large mass (bowel gas pattern eccentric, paucity of gas in one quadrant)
  fibroid ('popcorn' calcification).
- Ultrasound: ascites, may show cystic masses.
- CT scan: investigation of choice, differentiates origin and relationships.
- Paracentesis: MC+S (infections), cytology (tumours).
- Liver biopsy: undiagnosed hepatomegaly.

Key investigations—*abdominal wall swellings*

- Ultrasound: subcutaneous lumps.
- CT scan: abscesses, hernias.
- Herniography: rarely used for possible hernias with negative other investigations.
- Laparoscopy: diagnosis and possible treatment of hernia.

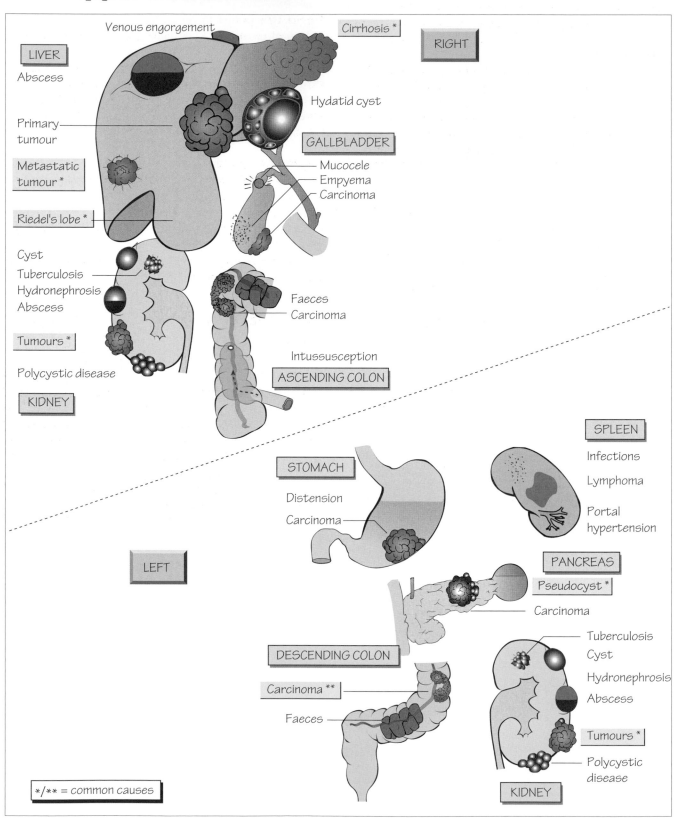

Venous engorgement

Cirrhosis *

RIGHT

LIVER

Abscess

Hydatid cyst

Primary
tumour

GALLBLADDER

Metastatic
tumour *

Mucocele
Empyema
Carcinoma

Riedel's lobe *

Cyst
Tuberculosis
Hydronephrosis
Abscess

Faeces
Carcinoma

Tumours *

Intussusception

Polycystic disease

ASCENDING COLON

KIDNEY

SPLEEN

Infections

STOMACH

Lymphoma

Distension

Portal
hypertension

Carcinoma

PANCREAS

LEFT

Pseudocyst *

Carcinoma

Tuberculosis
Cyst

DESCENDING COLON

Hydronephrosis

Abscess

Carcinoma **

Faeces

Tumours *

Polycystic
disease

*/** = common causes

KIDNEY

36 *Surgery at a Glance*, 4e. By P. Grace and N.R. Borley. Published 2009 by Blackwell Publishing. ISBN 978-1-4051-8325-3.

Liver

- Riedel's lobe: smooth, non-tender, lateral/right lobe:, 'tongue-like', men < women.
- Infective hepatitis: smooth, tender, global enlargement.
- Liver abscess: usually one large abscess, ?amoebic, very tender, systemically unwell.
- Hydatid cyst: smooth, may be loculated, ?history of tropical travel.
- Venous congestion: smooth, tender, pulsatile (slightly irregular (cirrhotic) if chronic).
- Cirrhosis: irregular, firm, 'knobbly'.
- Tumours:
  primary: solitary, large, non-tender, ?lobulated
  secondary: often multiple, irregular, rock hard, centrally umbilicated.

Gallbladder

- Generally: oval, smooth, projects towards RIF, beneath the tip of the ninth rib, moves with respiration.
- Mucocele: large gallbladder, moderately tender, smooth walled.
- Empyema: acutely tender, difficult to palpate clearly because of pain.

- Carcinoma of gallbladder: nodular, hard, irregular.
- Malignant obstruction of the lower end of the bile duct: palpable, painless, smooth gallbladder with jaundice.

Renal masses

- Perinephric abscess/pyonephrosis: acutely tender, systemic signs, rarely large.
- Hydronephrosis: large, smooth, tense kidney. May be massive.
- Solitary cyst: smooth, non-tender, may be massive.
- Polycystic disease: frequently very large, lobulated, smooth.
- Renal carcinoma: irregular, nodular, often hard, ?fixed.
- Nephroblastoma: large mass in children.

Suprarenal gland

- Generally: only palpable when large, moves with respiration, difficult to define borders.
- Adenomas: usually cystic if palpable.
- Infections: ?chronic fungal infections, may be tender, systemic features.
- Congenital hyperplasia: young children, endocrine disorders associated, smooth, non-tender.

Abdominal swellings (localized): upper abdominal/2

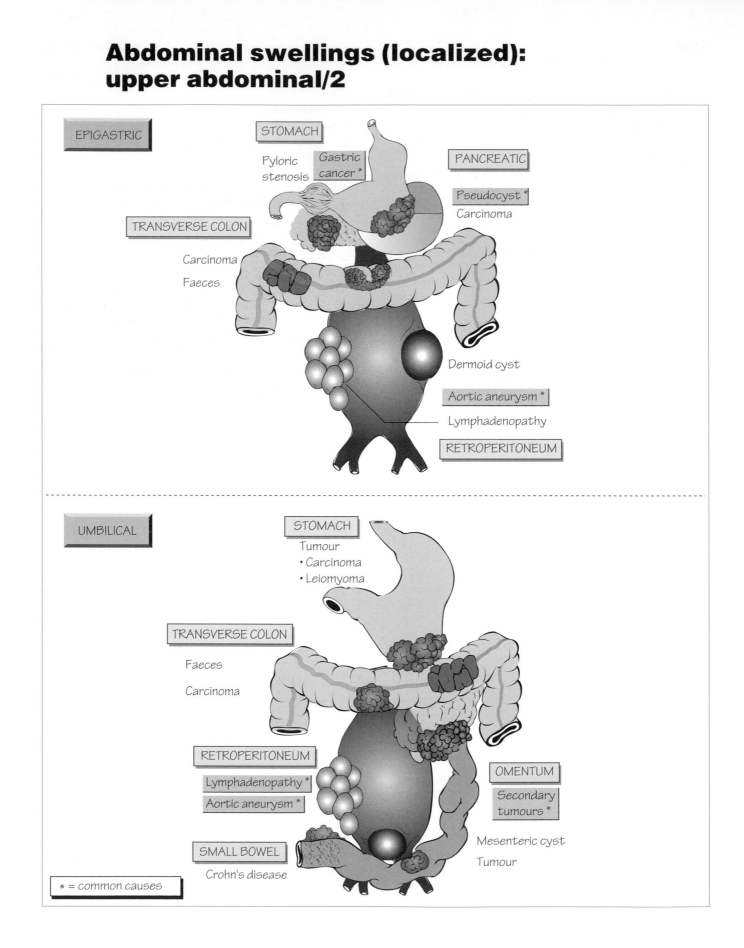

EPIGASTRIC

STOMACH

Pyloric stenosis

Gastric cancer *

PANCREATIC

Pseudocyst *

Carcinoma

TRANSVERSE COLON

Carcinoma

Faeces

Dermoid cyst

Aortic aneurysm *

Lymphadenopathy

RETROPERITONEUM

UMBILICAL

STOMACH

Tumour
• Carcinoma
• Leiomyoma

TRANSVERSE COLON

Faeces

Carcinoma

RETROPERITONEUM

Lymphadenopathy *

Aortic aneurysm *

OMENTUM

Secondary tumours *

Mesenteric cyst

Tumour

SMALL BOWEL

Crohn's disease

* = common causes

Colon

• Faeces: soft, putty-like mass, mobile, non-tender, can be indented.
• Carcinoma: firm-hard, irregular, non-tender, may be mobile (fixity strongly suggests carcinoma).
• Intussusception: mobile, smooth, sausage-shaped mass.

Stomach

• Gastric distension: soft, fluctuant, succussion splash present.
• Neoplasm: irregular, hard, craggy, immobile, does not descend on inspiration.

Pancreas

• Generally: does not move with respiration, fixed to retroperitoneum, poorly defined.
• Pseudocyst/cyst: mildly tender (worse if infected), symptoms of gastric obstruction.
• Carcinoma: hard, irregular, non-tender, fixed.

Retroperitoneum

• Lymphadenopathy: solid, immobile, irregular, 'rubbery', may be massive, particularly if lymphomatous.

• Dermoid cysts (rare): deep seated, smooth, recurrent after surgery.
• Aortic aneurysm: smooth, fusiform, pulsatile, expansile, may be tender.

Omentum

Secondary carcinoma: hard, irregular, mobile, 'pancake-like', often ovarian carcinoma.

Key investigations

• FBC: anaemia, tumours.
• WCC: lymphomas, Crohn's disease, appendicitis/diverticulitis.
• LFTs: liver lesions.
• Ultrasound: pancreatic (pseudo)cysts, aortic aneurysm.
• CT scan: pancreatic tumours, lymphadenopathy, retroperitoneal/mesenteric cysts, aortic aneurysm, omental deposits.
• Gastroscopy: stomach tumours.
• Colonoscopy: colonic tumours.
• Small bowel enema: small intestinal tumours.
• Barium enema: colonic tumours.

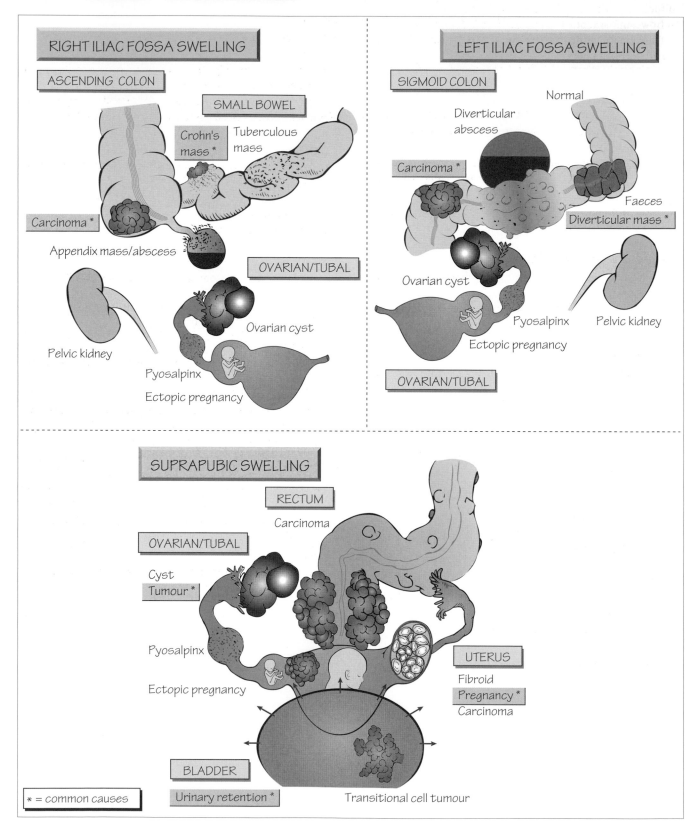

RIGHT ILIAC FOSSA SWELLING

ASCENDING COLON

SMALL BOWEL

Crohn's mass *

Tuberculous mass

Carcinoma *

Appendix mass/abscess

OVARIAN/TUBAL

Ovarian cyst

Pelvic kidney

Pyosalpinx

Ectopic pregnancy

LEFT ILIAC FOSSA SWELLING

SIGMOID COLON

Normal

Diverticular abscess

Carcinoma *

Faeces

Diverticular mass *

Ovarian cyst

Pyosalpinx

Pelvic kidney

Ectopic pregnancy

OVARIAN/TUBAL

SUPRAPUBIC SWELLING

RECTUM

Carcinoma

OVARIAN/TUBAL

Cyst
Tumour *

Pyosalpinx

Ectopic pregnancy

UTERUS

Fibroid
Pregnancy *
Carcinoma

BLADDER

* = common causes

Urinary retention *

Transitional cell tumour

Sigmoid colon

- Diverticular mass: tender, ill defined, rubbery hard, non-mobile.
- Paracolic abscess: acutely tender, ill defined, ?fluctuant, systemic upset.
- Carcinoma: hard, craggy, non-tender unless perforated, immobile, associated with altered bowel habit/obstructive symptoms.
- Faeces: firm, indentable/'malleable', mobile with colon.
- Normal: only in a thin person, non-tender, chord-like.

Caecum/ascending colon

- Appendix mass/abscess: acutely tender, ill defined, ?fluctuant, systemic upset.
- Carcinoma: hard, craggy, non-tender unless perforated, immobile, associated with anaemia/weight loss and anergia.

Terminal ileum

- Crohn's mass: tender, ill defined, rubbery hard, non-mobile.
- Tuberculous mass: mildly tender, ill defined, firm, associated with cutaneous sinuses, ?systemic TB.

Ovary/fallopian tube

- Cyst: may be massive, usually mobile, ?bimanually palpable on PV examination.
- Neoplasm.
- Ectopic pregnancy: very tender, associated with PV bleeding/intra-abdominal bleeding and collapse.
- Salpingo-oophoritis: very tender, bimanually palpable, associated with PV discharge.

Bladder

- Generally: midline swelling, extends up towards umbilicus, dull to percussion, non-mobile, cannot 'get below' it.
- Retention of urine: stony dull to percussion, associated with desire to pass urine, disappears on voiding/catheterization. May be no desire to pass urine with chronic retention.

- Transitional cell carcinoma: hard, irregular, fixed, may be associated with dysuria, haematuria and desire to pass urine on examination.

Uterus

- Pregnancy: smooth, regular, fetal heart sounds heard/movements.
- Fibromyoma: usually smooth, may be pedunculated and mobile, non-tender, associated menorrhagia.
- Uterine carcinoma: firm uterus, may be tender, irregular only if tumour is extrauterine, associated PV bloody discharge.

Rectum

Carcinoma: firm, irregular, non-tender, relatively immobile, associated alteration in bowel habit/PR bleeding.

Urachus (rare)

Cyst: small swelling in midline, ?associated umbilical discharge.

Other

Pelvic kidney: smooth, regular, non-tender, non-mobile.

Anatomy and normal bilirubin metabolism

New RBCs $\xrightarrow{\text{120 days}}$ Effete RBCs

Reticuloendothelial system
Hb → Haem

KIDNEY

Urobilinogen excreted in urine

Unconjugated bilirubin (water insoluble) bound to albumin

HEPATOCYTE
Bilirubin
↓ Glucuronyl transferase
Bilirubin glucuronide (conjugated bilirubin) (water soluble)

Enterohepatic circulation

SMALL BOWEL
Conjugated bilirubin
↓ Bacteria
Urobilinogen

Stercobilin excreted in faeces

Biochemical features of different types of jaundice

Type of jaundice	Haemolytic	Hepatocellular Early	Hepatocellular Late	Obstructive
Serum bilirubin				
Unconjugated	↑	N/↑	N/↑	N
Conjugated	N	N	↑	↑↑
Urinary bilirubin	N/↑	↑	↑	↑↑
Urobilinogen	N/↑	N	↓	↓↓
LFTs				
Alkaline phosphatase	N	N	↑	↑↑
γ-GT transaminase	N	↑	↑	↑↑
Transaminases	N	↑↑	↑↑	N/↑
Lactate dehydrogenase	N	↑↑	↑↑	N/↑
FBC				
Reticulocytes	> 2%	N	N	N

CAUSES OF OBSTRUCTIVE JAUNDICE

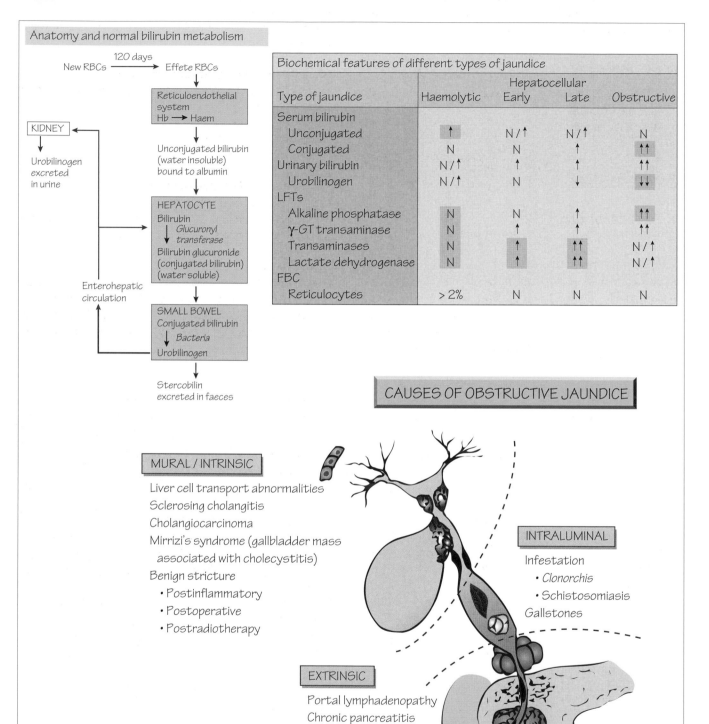

MURAL / INTRINSIC

Liver cell transport abnormalities
Sclerosing cholangitis
Cholangiocarcinoma
Mirrizi's syndrome (gallbladder mass associated with cholecystitis)
Benign stricture
• Postinflammatory
• Postoperative
• Postradiotherapy

INTRALUMINAL

Infestation
• Clonorchis
• Schistosomiasis
Gallstones

EXTRINSIC

Portal lymphadenopathy
Chronic pancreatitis
Pancreatic tumour
Ampullary tumour
Duodenal tumour

Definition

Jaundice (also called *icterus*) is defined as yellowing of the skin and sclera from accumulation of the pigment bilirubin in the blood and tissues. The bilirubin level has to exceed 35–40 mmol/L before jaundice is clinically apparent.

Key points

- Jaundice can be classified simply as pre-hepatic (haemolytic), hepatic (hepatocellular) and post-hepatic (obstructive).
- Most of the surgically treatable causes of jaundice are post-hepatic (obstructive).
- Painless progressive jaundice is highly likely to be due to malignancy.

Differential diagnosis

The following list explains the mechanisms behind the causes of jaundice.

Pre-hepatic/haemolytic jaundice
Haemolytic/congenital hyperbilirubinaemias

Excess production of unconjugated bilirubin exhausts the capacity of the liver to conjugate the extra load, e.g. haemolytic anaemias (e.g. hereditary spherocytosis, sickle cell disease, hypersplenism, thalassaemia).

Hepatic/hepatocellular jaundice
Hepatic unconjugated hyperbilirubinaemia

- Failure of transport of unconjugated bilirubin into the cell, e.g. Gilbert's syndrome.
- Failure of glucuronyl transferase activity, e.g. Crigler–Najjar syndrome.

Hepatic conjugated hyperbilirubinaemia

Hepatocellular injury. Hepatocyte injury results in failure of excretion of bilirubin:
- Infections: viral hepatitis.
- Poisons: CCl_4, aflatoxin.
- Drugs: paracetamol, halothane.

Post-hepatic/obstructive jaundice
Post-hepatic conjugated hyperbilirubinaemia

Anything that blocks the release of conjugated bilirubin from the hepatocyte or prevents its delivery to the duodenum.

Courvoisier's law

'A palpable gallbladder in the presence of jaundice is unlikely to be due to gallstones.' It usually indicates the presence of a neoplastic stricture (tumour of pancreas, ampulla, duodenum, CBD), chronic pancreatitic stricture or portal lymphadenopathy.

Key investigations

- FBC: haemolysis.
- LFTs: alkaline phosphatase (cholestasis), γ-GT and transaminases (hepatocellular).
- Clotting: PT (elevated in cholestatic and hepatocellular jaundice).
- Urinary urobilinogen

Haemolytic
- Blood film
- Reticulocyte count
- Autoantibody screen

Hepatocellular
- Viral titres: including hepatitis A/B/C, CMV, EBV
- Ultrasound: details of hepatic parenchyma.
- Liver biopsy: hepatocellular disease

Obstructive
U/S CBD and gallbladder

CBD dilated
No gallstones
↓
?Ca pancreas/CBD
↓
ERCP +/– stent
CT scan/MRCP

CBD dilated
Gallstones
↓
ERCP
Surgery

Other cause found
↓
ERCP
CT scan
↓
Surgery

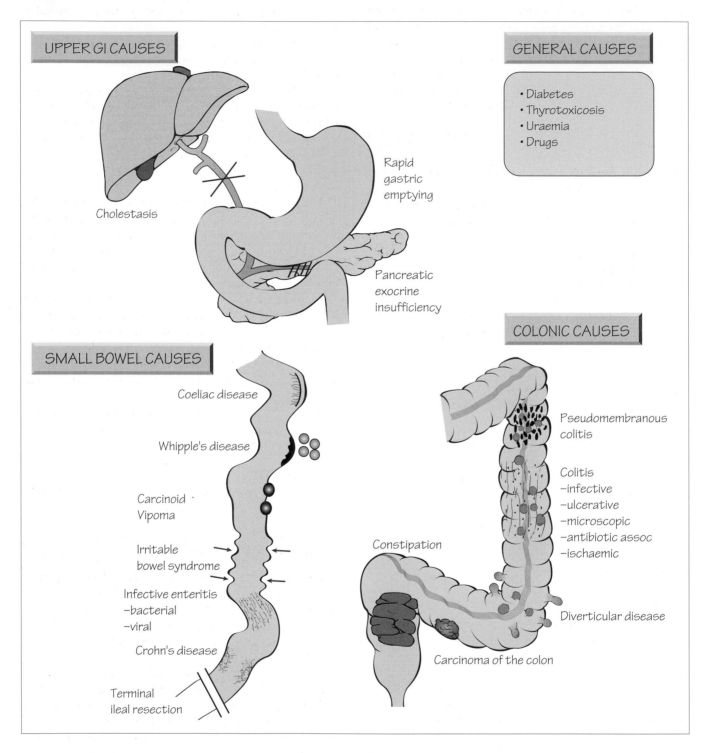

UPPER GI CAUSES

Cholestasis

Rapid gastric emptying

Pancreatic exocrine insufficiency

GENERAL CAUSES

- Diabetes
- Thyrotoxicosis
- Uraemia
- Drugs

SMALL BOWEL CAUSES

Coeliac disease

Whipple's disease

Carcinoid
Vipoma

Irritable bowel syndrome

Infective enteritis
–bacterial
–viral

Crohn's disease

Terminal ileal resection

COLONIC CAUSES

Pseudomembranous colitis

Colitis
–infective
–ulcerative
–microscopic
–antibiotic assoc
–ischaemic

Constipation

Diverticular disease

Carcinoma of the colon

44   *Surgery at a Glance*, 4e. By P. Grace and N.R. Borley. Published 2009 by Blackwell Publishing. ISBN 978-1-4051-8325-3.

Definitions

Diarrhoea is defined as the passage of loose, liquid stool. *Urgency* is the sensation of the need to defaecate without being able to delay. It may indicate rectal irritability but also occurs where the volume of liquid stool is too large, causing the rectum to be overwhelmed as a storage vessel. *Frequency* merely reflects the number of stools passed and may or may not be associated with urgency or diarrhoea. *Dysentery* is an infective, inflammatory disorder of the lower intestinal tract resulting in pain, severe diarrhoea and passage of blood and mucus per rectum.

Key points

- Bloody diarrhoea is always pathological and usually indicates colitis of one form or another.
- Infective causes are common in acute transient diarrhoea.
- In diarrhoea of uncertain origin, remember the endocrine causes.
- Consider parasitic/atypical bacterial infections in a history of foreign travel.
- Alternating morning diarrhoea and normal/pellety stools later in the day is rarely pathological.
- Diarrhoea developing in hospitalized patients may be due to *Clostridium difficile* infection—check for CD toxin in the stool.

Important diagnostic features
Acute diarrhoea
Infections

- Viral: rotavirus, enteric adenovirus, calcivirus (acute watery diarrhoea).
- Bacteria: *Vibrio cholera* (severe diarrhoea, 'rice water' stool, dehydration, history of foreign travel), *Shigella/Salmonella*, *Campylobacter*, *Yersinia* (bacterial dysentery—diarrhoea + blood + mucus), *Clostridium difficile* (green, offensive diarrhoea).
- Protozoa: *Giardia intestinalis*, *Cryptosporidium parvum* (watery diarrhoea), *Entamoeba histolytica* (occasionally diarrhoea + blood + mucus – amoebic dysentery).

Antibiotic related

Due to disruption of the normal colonic flora. Short-lived, self-limiting, mild colicky pain.

Pseudomembranous colitis

Most severe form of *Clostridium difficile* infection, characterized by severe diarrhoea which may be bloody but occasionally acute constipation may indicate severe disease. Characteristic features on colonoscopy ('baked bean'-like adherent mucopurulent pseudomembranes). Treatment is with oral metronidazole or vancomycin for 10 days.

Chronic diarrhoea
Small bowel disease

- Crohn's disease: diarrhoea, pain prominent, blood and mucus less common, young adults, long history, chronic malnourishment and weight loss.
- Coeliac disease: history of wheat and cereals intolerance, may present in adulthood with chronic diarrhoea and weight loss, abdominal pains.
- 'Blind loop' syndrome: frothy, foul-smelling liquid stool, due to bacterial overgrowth and fermentation, usually associated with previous surgery, may complicate Crohn's disease.
- Whipple's disease: tropheryma whipples, arthritis, malabsorption, diarrhoea, lymphadenopathy.

Large bowel disease

- Ulcerative colitis: intermittent, blood and mucus, colicky pains, young adults. May be a short history in first presentations. Rarely presents with acute fulminant colitis with acute abdominal signs.
- Colon cancer: older, occasional blood streaks and mucus, change in frequency may be the only feature, positive faecal occult blood, rectal mass.
- Ischaemic colitis: elderly, other evidence of cardiovascular disease; abdominal pain, fever, diarrhoea and rectal bleeding.
- Irritable bowel syndrome: diarrhoea and constipation mixed, bloating, colicky pain, small stool pellets, never blood.
- Spurious: impacted faeces in rectum, liquefied stool passes around faecal obstruction, elderly, mental illness, constipating drugs.
- Polyps (villous) (rare): watery, mucoid diarrhoea, K^+ loss, most common in rectum.
- Diverticular disease (rare).

Systemic disease

Thyrotoxicosis, anxiety, peptides from tumours (VIP, serotonin, substance P, calcitonin), laxative abuse.

Key investigations

- FBC: leucocytosis (infective causes, colitis), anaemia (colon cancer, ulcerative colitis, diverticular disease).
- Anti α-gliadin Abs TTG lutaminase: coeliac disease.
- Thyroid function tests: hyperthyroidism.
- Stool culture: infections (remember microscopy for parasites).
- Proctoscopy/sigmoidoscopy: cancer, colitis, polyps (simple, easy, cheap and safe; performed in outpatients).
- Flexible sigmoidoscopy: cancer, polyps, colitis, infections (relatively safe, well tolerated, high sensitivity).
- Colonoscopy: colitis (extent and severity), pseudomembranous colitis.
- Small bowel enema: Crohn's disease, coeliac disease, Whipple's disease.
- Faecal elastase, faecal fat estimation/ERCP: pancreatic insufficiency.

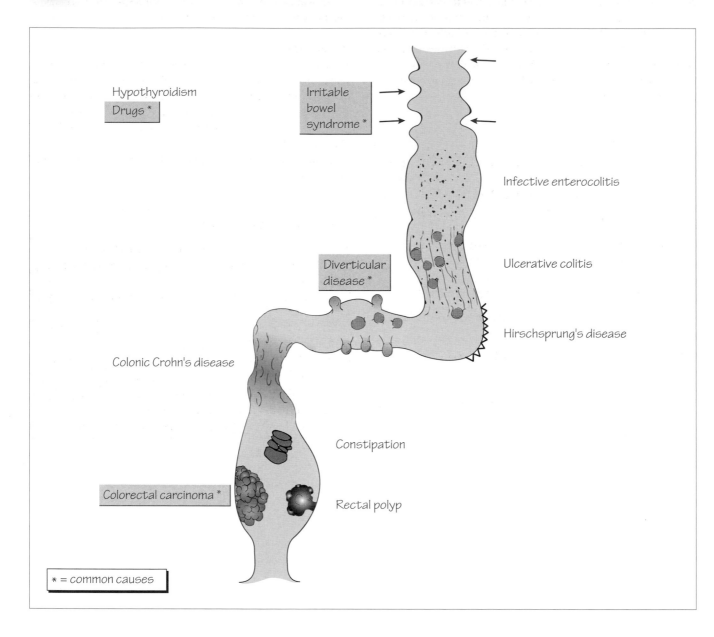

Hypothyroidism
Drugs *

Irritable bowel syndrome *

Infective enterocolitis

Diverticular disease *

Ulcerative colitis

Hirschsprung's disease

Colonic Crohn's disease

Constipation

Colorectal carcinoma *

Rectal polyp

* = common causes

Definitions

'Normal' bowel habit varies widely from person to person. Alterations in bowel habit are common manifestations of GI disease. *Constipation* is defined as infrequent or difficult evacuation of faeces and can be acute or chronic. *Absolute constipation* is defined as the inability to pass either faeces or flatus. *Diarrhoea* is an increase in the fluidity of stool. *Tenesmus* is the sensation of incomplete or unsatisfactory evacuation, often with rectal pain/discomfort.

Key points

- Acute constipation often indicates intestinal obstruction. The cardinal symptoms of obstruction are colicky abdominal pain, vomiting, constipation and distension.
- Chronic constipation may be a lifelong problem or may develop slowly in later life.
- All alterations in bowel habit that persist must be investigated for an underlying cause—colorectal neoplasms are common causes, especially in the elderly.
- IBS is a diagnosis of exclusion and should rarely be considered for new symptoms age >55.

Important diagnostic features
Chronic constipation
Bowel disease

- Colon cancer: gradual onset, colicky abdominal pain, associated weight loss, anergia, anaemia, positive faecal occult bloods, abdominal mass.

- Diverticular disease: associated LIF pains, inflammatory episodes, rectal bleeding.
- Perianal pain, e.g. fissure, perianal abscess—due to spasm of the internal anal sphincter, common in children.

Adynamic bowel

- Hirschsprung's disease: constipation from birth, gross abdominal distension. Short-segment Hirschprung's disease (involving only the lower rectum) may present in adulthood with worsening chronic constipation and megarectum/megasigmoid.
- Drugs: opiates, anticholinergics, antipsychotics, secondary to chronic laxative abuse.
- Pregnancy: due to progesterone effects on smooth muscle of bowel wall.

Key investigations

- Rectal examination: rectal cancer, rectal adenoma.
- FBC: anaemia from colon cancer, ulcerative colitis, diverticular disease.
- Stool culture: infections (remember microscopy for parasites).
- Proctoscopy/sigmoidoscopy: cancer, colitis, polyps (simple, easy, cheap and safe; performed in outpatients).
- Flexible sigmoidoscopy: cancer, polyps, colitis, infections (relatively safe, well tolerated, high sensitivity).
- Barium enema: best for tumours of proximal colon.
- Colonoscopy: colitis (extent and severity).
- Rectal biopsy (full thickness): Hirschprung's disease.

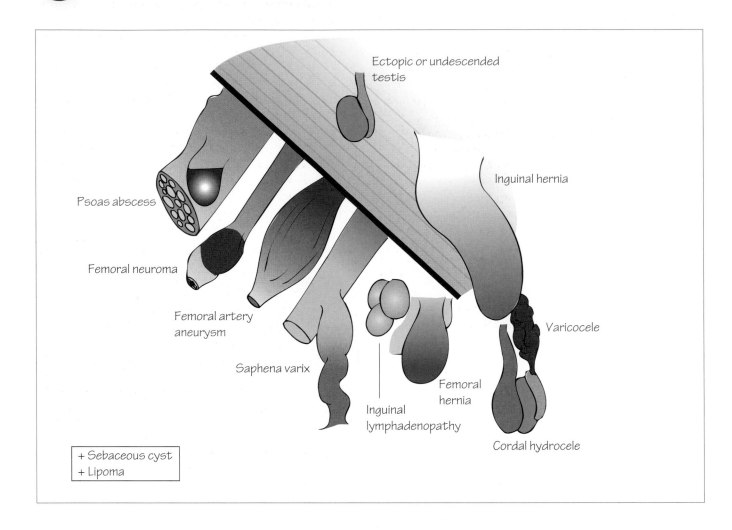

Ectopic or undescended testis

Psoas abscess

Femoral neuroma

Femoral artery aneurysm

Saphena varix

Inguinal lymphadenopathy

Femoral hernia

Inguinal hernia

Varicocele

Cordal hydrocele

+ Sebaceous cyst
+ Lipoma

Definition

Any swelling in the inguinal area or upper medial thigh.

Key points

- The groin crease does not mark the inguinal ligament in most people and is an unreliable landmark.
- Inguinal hernias are common, always start above and medial to the pubic tubercle, may be medial or lateral to it and usually emphasize the groin crease on that side.
- Femoral hernias always start below and lateral to the pubic tubercle and usually flatten the skin crease on that side.
- Femoral hernias are more common in women, are high risk and need urgent attention.
- Masses in the groin and scrotum together are inguinal hernias.
- Inguinal lymphadenopathy may be isolated or may be part of systemic lymphadenopathy. A cause should always be sought.

Important diagnostic features

The types, causes and features are listed below.

Inguinal hernia

- Direct inguinal hernia: not controlled by pressure over internal ring, characteristically causes a 'forward' bulge in the groin, does not descend into the scrotum.
- Indirect inguinal hernia: controlled by pressure over internal ring, 'slides' through the inguinal canal, often descends into the scrotum.
- Undescended testis: often mass at the external ring or inguinal canal, associated with hypoplastic hemi-scrotum, frequently associated with indirect inguinal hernia.
- Spermatic cord: 'cordal' hydrocele, does not have a cough impulse, may be possible to define upper edge, fluctuates and transilluminates.
- Lipoma: soft, fleshy, does not transilluminate or fluctuate.

Femoral hernia

- Femoral hernia: elderly women (mostly), may be tender and non-expansile, not reducible, groin crease often lost, high risk of strangulation and obstruction.
- Saphena varix: expansile, cough impulse, thrill on percussion of distal saphenous vein.
- Lymphadenopathy: hard, discrete nodules, often multiple or an indistinct mass.
- Femoral artery aneurysm: expansile, pulsatile, thrill and bruit may be present.
- Psoas abscess (rare): soft, fluctuant and compressible, lateral to the femoral artery, may be 'cold' abscesses caused by TB.
- Femoral neuroma (very rare): hard, smooth, moves laterally but not vertically, pressure may cause pain in the distribution of the femoral nerve.
- Hydrocele of femoral sac (very very rare).

Key investigations

- FBC: causes of lymphadenopathy.
- Ultrasound: femoral aneurysm, saphena varix, psoas abscess, ectopic testicle. Also sometimes useful to identify small femoral hernias.
- CT scan: cause of psoas abscess.
- Herniography: rarely needed to confirm presence of hernia if operative indication not clear.
- Laparoscopy: may be used as both diagnostic and therapeutic manoeuvre.

Principles of hernia surgery

- Femoral hernia: close the canal only (usually sutured—may be mesh 'plug' if large defect).
- Infantile inguinal hernia: excise/close the sac only ('herniotomy'). No repair of the canal is required. Do not use mesh.
- Adult inguinal hernia:
  reduce the sac and its contents (sac excision not necessary)
  reinforce the canal without tension (usually mesh)
  surgical approach may be open (transcutaneous) under GA or LA or laparoscopic (extra-/pre-peritoneal, transperitoneal)—always GA.

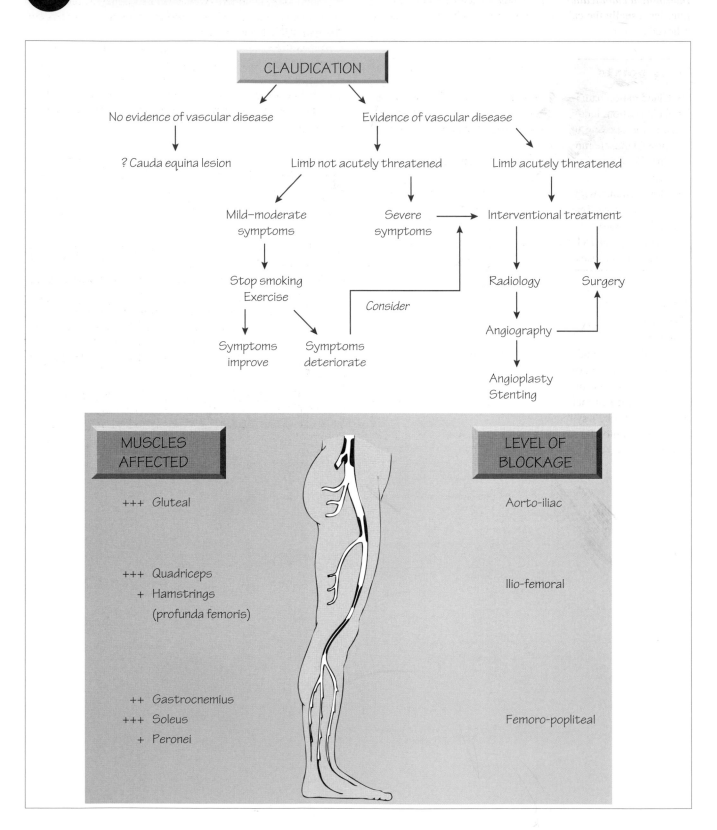

CLAUDICATION

No evidence of vascular disease → ? Cauda equina lesion

Evidence of vascular disease → Limb not acutely threatened / Limb acutely threatened

Limb not acutely threatened → Mild–moderate symptoms → Stop smoking Exercise → Symptoms improve / Symptoms deteriorate

Limb not acutely threatened → Severe symptoms → Interventional treatment

Limb acutely threatened → Interventional treatment

Consider

Interventional treatment → Radiology → Angiography → Angioplasty Stenting

Interventional treatment → Surgery

Angiography → Surgery

MUSCLES AFFECTED

+++ Gluteal

+++ Quadriceps
  + Hamstrings
    (profunda femoris)

 ++ Gastrocnemius
+++ Soleus
  + Peronei

LEVEL OF BLOCKAGE

Aorto-iliac

Ilio-femoral

Femoro-popliteal

Definition

Intermittent claudication is defined as an aching pain in the leg muscles, usually the calf, that is precipitated by walking and is relieved by rest.

Key points

- Claudication pain is always reversible and relieved by rest.
- Claudication tends to improve with time and exercise due to the opening up of new collateral supply vessels and improved muscle function.
- The site of disease is one level higher than the highest level of affected muscles.
- Most patients with claudication have associated vascular disease and investigation for occult coronary or cerebrovascular is mandatory.
- Cauda equina ischaemia caused by osteoarthritis of the spine can also cause intermittent claudication.

Differential diagnosis

Vascular

Atheroma

- Typical patient: male, over 45 years, ischaemic heart disease, smoker, diabetic, overweight.
- Aortic occlusion: buttock, thigh and possibly calf claudication, impotence in males, absent femoral pulses and below in both legs (Leriche's syndrome).
- Iliac or common femoral stenosis: thigh and calf claudication, absent/weak femoral pulses in affected limb.

- Femoro-popliteal stenosis: calf claudication only, absent popliteal and distal pulses.

Neurological

Cauda equina

Elderly patients, atypical history, history of chronic back pain or back injury, pain may be bilateral and in the distribution of the S1–S3 dermatomes, may be accompanied by paraesthesia in the feet and loss of ankle jerks, all peripheral pulses palpable and legs well perfused.

Key investigations

- FBC: exclude polycythaemia.
- Glucose: diabetes.
- Lipids: hyperlipidaemia.
- ABI: (pre and post exercise) estimate of disease severity.
- ECG: coronary disease.
- Angiography: precise location and extent of disease, pre-procedure planning.
  catheter angiography: a catheter is inserted into the artery and contrast given intra-arterially, standard or digital substraction X-ray images obtained—invasive
  CT angiography: IV contrast given and CT images obtained
  MRA: IV contrast given (Gadolinium), MR images obtained—no radiation.
- Duplex ultrasound scanning sometimes used instead of angiography.

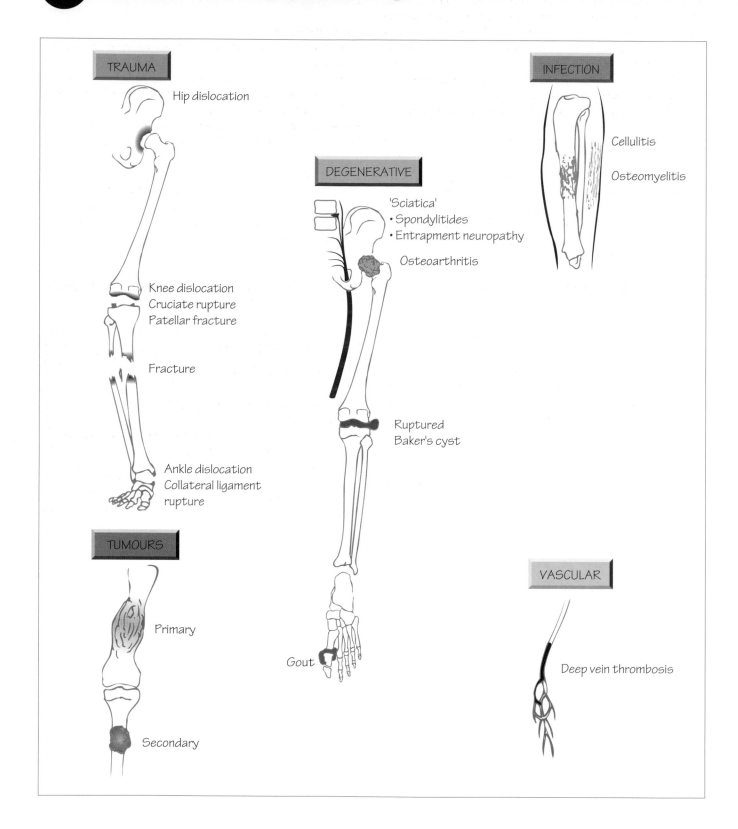

TRAUMA

Hip dislocation

Knee dislocation
Cruciate rupture
Patellar fracture

Fracture

Ankle dislocation
Collateral ligament
rupture

TUMOURS

Primary

Secondary

DEGENERATIVE

'Sciatica'
• Spondylitides
• Entrapment neuropathy

Osteoarthritis

Ruptured
Baker's cyst

Gout

INFECTION

Cellulitis

Osteomyelitis

VASCULAR

Deep vein thrombosis

Definitions

Acute leg pain is a subjective, unpleasant sensation felt somewhere in the lower limb. *Referred pain* is the perception of pain in an area remote from the site of origin of the pain, e.g. leg pain from lumbar disc herniation, knee pain from hip pathology. *Cramps* are involuntary, painful contractions of voluntary muscles. *Sciatica* is a nerve pain caused by irritation of the sciatic nerve roots characterized by lumbosacral pain radiating down the back of the thigh, lateral side of the calf and into the foot.

> ## Key points
>
> - May be due to pathology arising in any of the tissues of the leg.
> - Constant or lasting pain suggests local pathology.
> - Transient or intermittent pain suggests referred pathology.
> - Systemic symptoms or upset suggests inflammation.

Important diagnostic features

Infection

- Infection of skin (cellulitis): painful, swollen, red, hot leg, associated systemic features—pyrexia, rigors, anorexia, commonly caused by *Streptococcus pyogenes*. May be associated lymphangitis (inflammation of lymphatics).
- Acute osteomyelitis: staphylococcal infection, affects metaphyses, acute pain, tenderness and oedema over the end of a long bone, common in children, may be history of skin infection or trauma.

Trauma

- Muscle: swollen, tender and painful, pain worse on attempted movement of the affected muscle.
- Bone: painful, tender. Swelling, deformity, discoloration, bruising and crepitus suggest fracture.
- Joints: painful, limited movement, deformity if dislocated, locking and instability with knee injury.

Degenerative

- Gout: first MTP joint (big toe), males, associated signs of joint inflammation.
- Disc herniation (sciatica): pain in distribution of one or two nerve roots, sudden onset, back pain and stiffness, lumbar scoliosis due to muscle spasm.
- Ruptured Baker's cyst: pain mostly behind the knee, previous history of knee arthritis, calf may be hot and swollen.

Tumours

Bone: deep pain, worse in morning and after exercise, overlying muscle tenderness, pathological fractures, primary (e.g. osteosarcoma, osteoclastoma) or secondary (e.g. breast, prostate, lung metastasis).

Vascular

DVT: calf pain, swelling, redness, prominent superficial veins, tender on calf compression, low-grade pyrexia.

> ## Key investigations
>
> - FBC: WCC in infection.
> - D-Dimers: suspected DVT.
> - Blood cultures: spreading cellulitis.
> - Clotting: DVT.
> - Plain X-ray: trauma, osteomyelitis, bone tumours, gout.
> - MRI: suspected disc herniation.
> - Duplex ultrasound: DVT.
> - Venography: rarely used now as duplex ultrasound is as good, non-invasive and widely available.

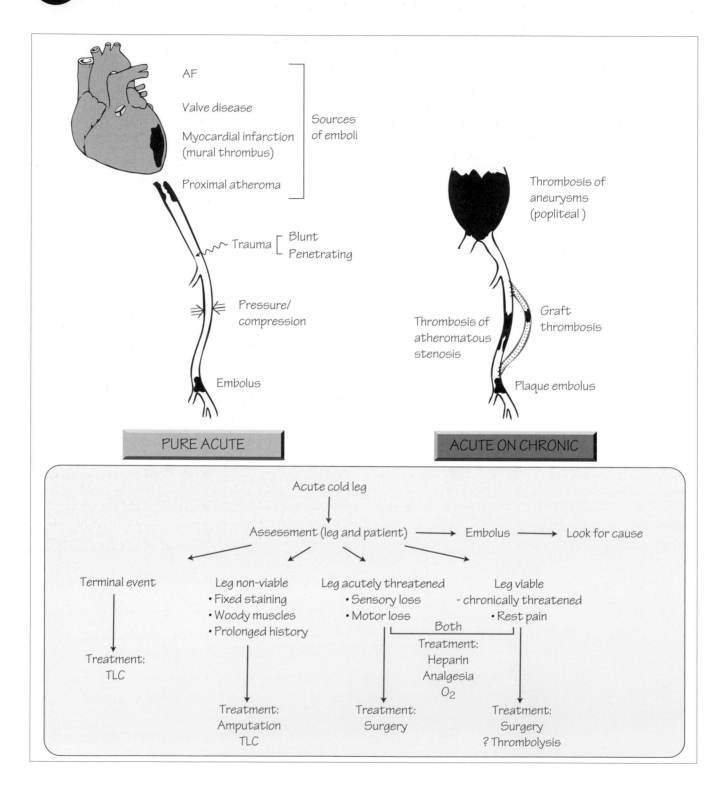

AF

Valve disease

Myocardial infarction
(mural thrombus)

Proximal atheroma

Sources
of emboli

Trauma [Blunt
Penetrating

Pressure/
compression

Embolus

Thrombosis of
aneurysms
(popliteal)

Thrombosis of
atheromatous
stenosis

Graft
thrombosis

Plaque embolus

PURE ACUTE

ACUTE ON CHRONIC

Acute cold leg

Assessment (leg and patient) → Embolus → Look for cause

Terminal event

Treatment:
TLC

Leg non-viable
• Fixed staining
• Woody muscles
• Prolonged history

Treatment:
Amputation
TLC

Leg acutely threatened
• Sensory loss
• Motor loss

Leg viable
- chronically threatened

• Rest pain

Both

Treatment:
Heparin
Analgesia
O_2

Treatment:
Surgery

Treatment:
Surgery
? Thrombolysis

Definition

The 'acute cold leg' is a clinical syndrome of the sudden onset of symptoms indicative of the presence of ischaemia sufficient to threaten the viability of the limb or part of it.

Key points

- Remember the '6 Ps' of acute ischaemia—pain, pallor, paraesthesia, paralysis, pulselessness, perishing cold.
- An acute cold leg is a surgical emergency and requires prompt diagnosis and treatment.
- 80% of acute cold legs presenting as an emergency have underlying chronic vascular pathology.
- Fasciotomies should always be considered as part of treatment if a leg is being revascularized.

Important diagnostic features

Isolated arterial embolus

- Sudden-onset severe ischaemia, no previous symptoms of vascular disease, previous history of atrial fibrillation/recent myocardial infarction, all peripheral pulses on the unaffected limb normal (suggesting no underlying PVD).
- Limb usually acutely threatened due to complete occlusion with no collateral supply.
- Common sites of impaction are: popliteal bi(tri)furcation, distal superficial femoral artery (adductor canal), origin of the profunda femoris. 'Saddle' embolus at aortic bifurcation causes bilateral acute ischaemic limbs.

Trauma

- May be due to direct injury to the vessel or by secondary compression due to bone fragments or haematoma.
- Direct injuries may be due to complete division of the vessel, distraction injury, damage and *in situ* thrombosis, foreign body, false aneurysm.

Thrombosis (*in situ*)

- Usually associated with underlying atheroma predisposing to thrombosis after minor trauma or immobility (after a fall or illness).
- May be subacute in onset, previous history of known vascular disease or intermittent claudication, associated risk factors for peripheral vascular disease, abnormal pulses in the unaffected limb.
- Paradoxically, the limb may not be as acutely threatened as in isolated arterial embolus because collateral vessels may already be present due to underlying disease.

Graft thrombosis

Often subacute in onset, limb not acutely threatened, progressive symptoms, loss of graft pulsation.

Aneurysm thrombosis

- Most common site—popliteal aneurysms.
- Sudden-onset limb ischaemia, acutely threatened, may be associated embolization as well, non-pulsatile mass in popliteal fossa, many have contralateral asymptomatic popliteal aneurysm.

Key investigations

- FBC: polycythaemia.
- U+E: renal impairment, myonecrosis.
- Clotting: thrombophilia.
- ECG, ECHO: atrial fibrillation, myocardial infarction, valve disease.
- Duplex scanning: graft patency, popliteal aneurysm.
- Angiography: wherever possible—arterial embolism, thrombosis, underlying PVD.

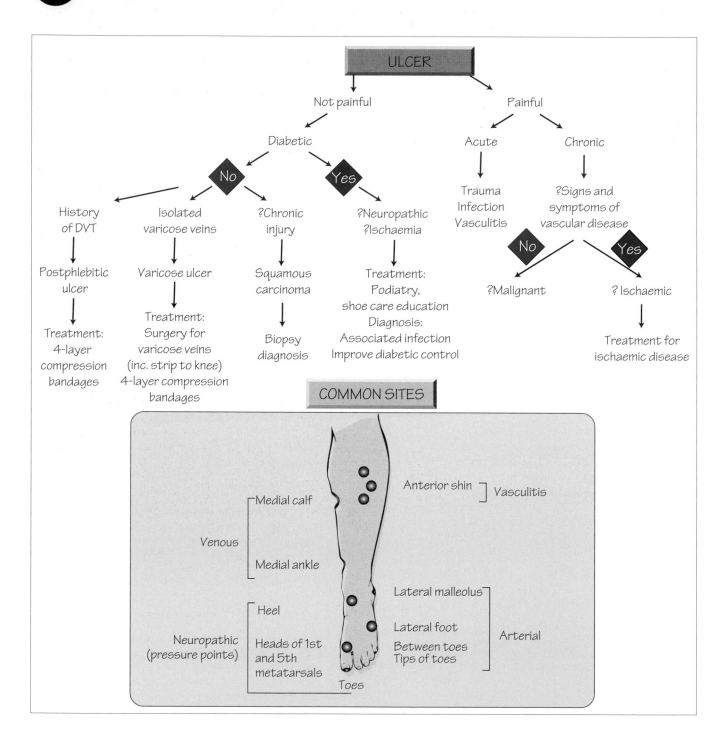

Definition

An *ulcer* is defined as an area of discontinuity of the surface epithelium. A *leg ulcer* is an area of ulceration anywhere on the lower limb but usually sited below the knee or on the foot.

> ### Key points
>
> • Pain suggests ischaemia or infection.
> • Neuropathic ulcers occur over points of pressure and trauma.
> • Marked worsening of a chronic ulcer suggests malignant change.
> • The underlying cause must be treated first or the ulcer will not heal.
> • Several precipitating causes may coexist (e.g. diabetes, PVD and neuropathy).
> • If underlying varicose veins are present with a venous ulcer they should be treated.

Important diagnostic features
Venous ulcers

• Venous hypertension secondary to DVT or varicose veins: ulceration on the medial side of the leg, above the ankle, any size, shallow with sloping edges, bleeds after minor trauma, weeps readily, associated dermato-liposclerosis.
• If deep venous disease is suspected duplex scanning of the veins is indicated.

Arterial ulcers

Occlusive arterial disease: painful ulcers, do not bleed, non-healing, lateral ankle, heel, metatarsal heads, tips of the toes, associated features of ischaemia, e.g. claudication, absent pulses, pallor. Elderly patients may present with 'blue toe' syndrome which is caused by microemboli.

Diabetic ulcers

• Ischaemic: same as arterial ulcers.
• Neuropathic: deep, painless ulcers, plantar aspect of foot or toes, associated with cellulitis, deep tissue abscesses, oedema, warm foot, pulses may be present.

Malignant ulcers

• Squamous cell carcinoma: may arise *de novo* or malignant change in a chronic ulcer or burn (Marjolin's ulcer). Large ulcer, heaped up, everted edges. Lymphadenopathy—highly suspicious.
• Basal cell carcinoma: uncommon on the leg, rolled edges, pearly white.
• Malignant melanoma: lower limb is a common site, consider malignant if increase in size or pigmentation, bleeding, itching or ulceration.

Miscellaneous ulcers

• Trauma: may be caused by minor trauma. Predisposing factors are poor circulation, malnutrition or steroid treatment.
• Vasculitis (rare), e.g. rheumatoid arthritis, SLE.
• Infections (rare): syphilis, TB, tropical infections.
• Pyoderma gangrenosum: multiple necrotic ulcers over the legs that start as nodules. Seen with ulcerative colitis and Crohn's disease.

> ### Key investigations
>
> • FBC: infections.
> • Glucose: diabetes.
> • Special blood tests: TPHA (syphilis), ANCA (SLE), Rh factor.
> • ABI measurement to exclude underlying PVD. Toe pressures more accurate in diabetes.
> • Doppler ultrasound: assessment of venous disease, assessment of arterial disease (above the knee). Simple, cheap, highly sensitive, good screening test.
> • Biopsy: malignancy. Melanoma—always excision biopsy. Others may be incision/'punch'.
> • Duplex ultrasound/angiography/(rarely venography)/: extent and severity of disease. Planning treatment.

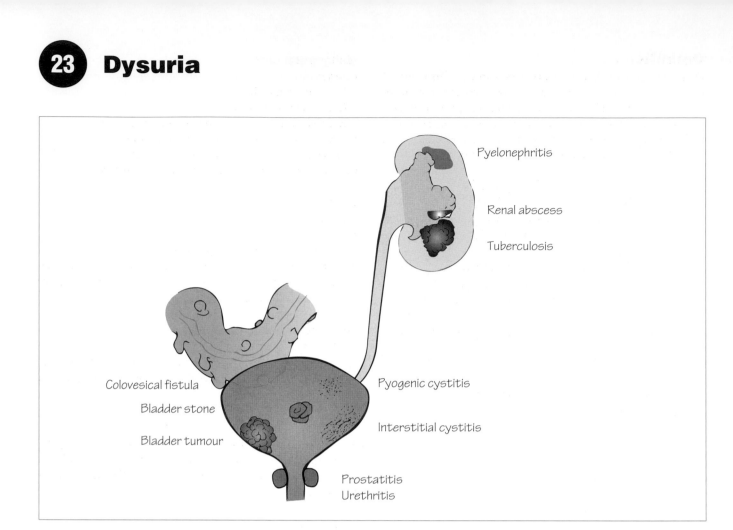

Pyelonephritis

Renal abscess

Tuberculosis

Co   Pyogenic cystitis
Colovesical fistula

Bladder stone   Interstitial cystitis

Bladder tumour

Prostatitis
Urethritis

Definitions

Dysuria is defined as a pain that arises from an irritation of the urethra and is felt during micturition. *Frequency* indicates increased passage of urine during the daytime; *nocturia* indicates increased passage of urine during the night. *Urgency* is an uncontrollable desire to micturate and may be associated with *incontinence*, which is the involuntary loss of urine.

Key points

- UTI is the most common cause of dysuria in adults.
- Systemic upset and loin pain suggest an ascending UTI (pyelonephritis).
- Elderly men with recurrent UTIs often have an underlying problem of bladder emptying due to prostate disease.
- Recurrent infections require investigation to exclude an underlying cause.
- Pneumaturia, 'bits' in the urine and coliform infections suggest a colovesical fistula.

Important diagnostic features

Urinary tract infection

Acute pyelonephritis

Cause: Upper tract infection.

Predisposing causes:

- Outflow tract obstruction.
- Vesicoureteric reflux.
- Renal or bladder calculi.
- Diabetes mellitus.
- Neuropathic bladder dysfunction.

Features: Pyrexia, rigors, flank pain, dysuria, malaise, anorexia, leucocytosis, pyuria (>10 WBC/mm^3 urine), bacteriuria, microscopic haematuria, C&S >100 000 organisms/mL. Steile pyuria may be caused by perinephric abscess, urethral syndrome, chronic prostatitis, renal TB and fungal infections.

Acute cystitis

Causes:

- Lower tract infection.
- Usually coliform bacteria.
- Because of short urethra more common in females.
- *Proteus* infections may indicate stone disease.

Features: Dysuria, frequency, urgency, suprapubic pain, low back pain, incontinence and microscopic haematuria.

Urethritis

Causes:

- Sexually transmitted diseases.
- May be gonococcal, chlamydial or mycoplasmal.

Features: Dysuria and meatal pruritus, occurs 3–10 days after sexual contact, yellowish purulent urethral discharge suggests *Gonococcus*, thin mucoid discharge suggests *Chlamydia*.

Other causes of dysuria

Urethral syndrome

A condition characterized by frequency, urgency and dysuria in women with urine cultures showing no growth or low bacterial counts.

Vaginitis

A condition characterized by dysuria, pruritus and vaginal discharge. Urine cultures are negative, but vaginal cultures often reveal *Trichomonas vaginalis*, *Candida albicans* or *Haemophilus vaginalis*.

Bladder problems

- Bladder tumours are an uncommon cause of dysuria (10%), they usually present with haematuria.
- Interstitial cystitis: a chronic inflammatory condition of the bladder that causes frequent, urgent and painful urination with or without pelvic discomfort.
- Colovesical fistula: usually caused by diverticular disease.

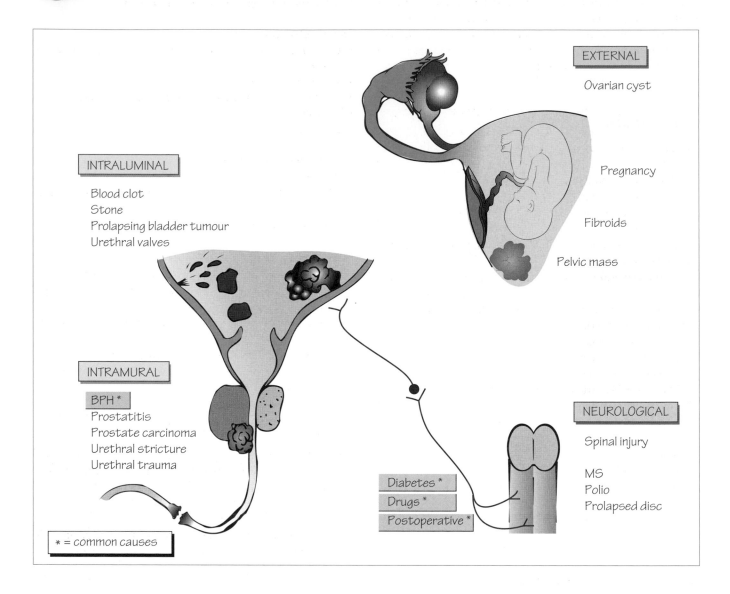

INTRALUMINAL

Blood clot
Stone
Prolapsing bladder tumour
Urethral valves

INTRAMURAL

BPH *
Prostatitis
Prostate carcinoma
Urethral stricture
Urethral trauma

* = common causes

EXTERNAL

Ovarian cyst

Pregnancy

Fibroids

Pelvic mass

NEUROLOGICAL

Spinal injury

MS
Polio
Prolapsed disc

Diabetes *
Drugs *
Postoperative *

Definitions

Urinary retention is defined as an inability to micturate (pass urine). *Acute urinary retention* is the sudden inability to micturate in the presence of a painful bladder. *Chronic urinary retention* is the presence of an enlarged, full, painless bladder with or without difficulty in micturition. *Overflow incontinence* is an uncontrollable leakage and dribbling of urine from the urethra in the presence of a full bladder.

Key points

Acute retention: characterized by pain, sensation of bladder fullness and a mildly distended bladder.

Remember common causes:
- Children—abdominal pain, drugs.
- Young—postoperative, drugs, acute UTI, trauma, haematuria.
- Elderly—acute on chronic retention with BPH, tumours, postoperative.

Chronic retention: characterized by symptoms of bladder irritation (frequency, dysuria, small volume), or painless, marked distension, overflow incontinence (often associated with secondary UTI).

Remember common causes:
- Children—congenital abnormalities.
- Young—trauma, postoperative.
- Elderly—BPH, strictures, prostatic carcinoma.

Neurogenic retention:
- Upper motor neurone causes produce chronic retention with reflex incontinence.
- Lower motor neurone causes produce chronic retention with overflow incontinence.
- Urinary retention is uncommon in young adults and almost always requires investigation to exclude underlying cause.
- Retention is common in elderly men—often due to prostate pathology.

Differential diagnosis

Mechanical

In the lumen of the urethra

- Congenital valves (rare): neonates, males, recurrent UTIs.
- Foreign body (rare).

- Stones (rare): acute pain in penis and glans.
- Tumour (rare): TCC or squamous cell carcinoma, history of haematuria, working in dye or rubber industry.

In the wall of the urethra

- BPH: frequency, nocturia, hesitancy, poor stream, dribbling, urgency.
- Tumour: as above.
- Stricture: history of trauma or serious infection, gradual onset of poor stream.
- Trauma: blood at meatus.

Outside the wall of the urethra

- Pregnancy.
- Fibroids: palpable, bulky uterus, menorrhagia, dysmenorrhoea.
- Ovarian cyst: mobile iliac fossa mass.
- Faecal impaction: spurious diarrhoea.

Neurological

- Postoperative: pain, drugs, pelvic nerve disturbance.
- Spinal cord injuries: acute phase is lower motor neurone type, late phase is upper motor neurone type.
- Drugs: narcotics, anticholinergics, antihistamines, antipsychotics.
- Diabetes: progressive lower motor neurone pattern.
- Idiopathic: detrusor sphincter dyssynergia, ?bladder neurone degeneration.

Key investigations

- U+E: renal function.
- MSU MC+S: associated infection, include cytology where tumour suspected.
- Cystography: urethral valves, strictures.
- IVU: renal/bladder stones.
- Urodynamics: allows identification and assessment of neurological problems, assesses BPH.
- Cystoscopy.

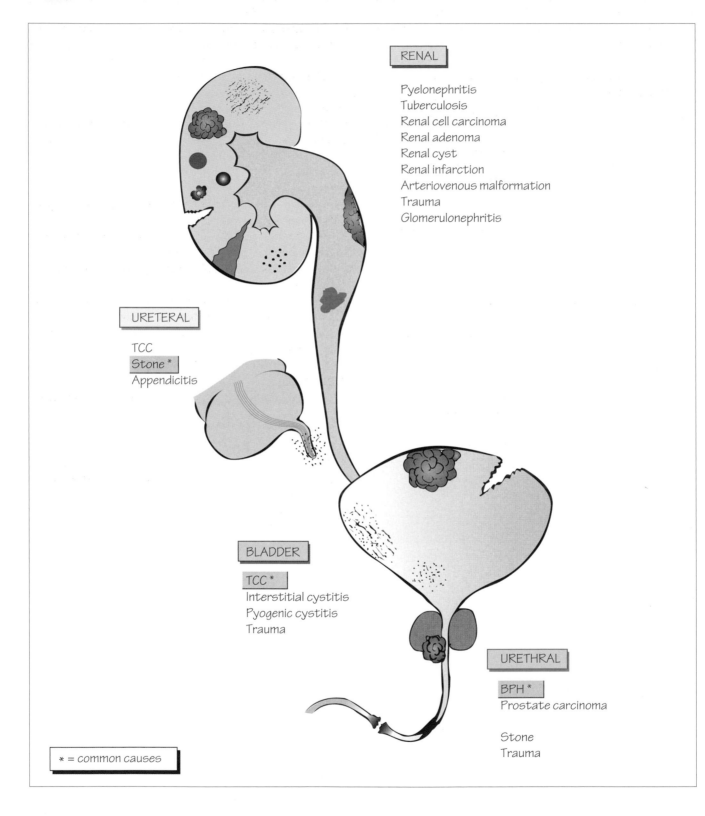

RENAL

Pyelonephritis
Tuberculosis
Renal cell carcinoma
Renal adenoma
Renal cyst
Renal infarction
Arteriovenous malformation
Trauma
Glomerulonephritis

URETERAL

TCC
Stone *
Appendicitis

BLADDER

TCC *
Interstitial cystitis
Pyogenic cystitis
Trauma

URETHRAL

BPH *
Prostate carcinoma

Stone
Trauma

* = common causes

Definitions

Haematuria is the passage of blood in the urine. *Frank haematuria* is the presence of blood on macroscopic examination, while *microscopic haematuria* indicates that RBCs are only seen on microscopy. *Haemoglobinuria* is defined as the presence of free Hb in the urine.

Key points

- Haematuria always requires investigation to exclude an underlying cause.
- Initial haematuria (blood on commencing urination) suggests a urethral cause.
- Terminal haematuria (blood after passing urine) suggests a bladder base or prostatic cause.
- Ribbon clots suggest a pelvi-ureteric cause.
- Renal bleeding can mimic colic due to clots passing down the ureter.

Important diagnostic features

Kidney

- Trauma: mild to moderate trauma commonly causes renal bleeding, severe injuries may not bleed (avulsed kidney—complete disruption).
- Tumours: may be profuse or intermittent.
- Renal cell carcinoma: associated mass, loin pain, clot colic or fever, occasional polycythaemia, hypercalcaemia and hypertension.
- TCC: characteristically painless, intermittent haematuria.
- Calculus: severe loin/groin pain, gross or microscopic, associated infection.
- Glomerulonephritis: usually microscopic, associated systemic disease (e.g. SLE).
- Pyelonephritis (rare).
- Renal tuberculosis (rare): sterile pyuria, weight loss, anorexia, PUO, increased frequency of micturition day and night.
- Polycystic disease (rare): palpable kidneys, hypertension, chronic renal failure.
- Renal arteriovenous malformation or simple cyst (very rare): painless, no other symptoms.
- Renal infarction (very rare): may be caused by an arterial embolus, painful tender kidney.

Ureter

- Calculus: severe loin/groin pain, gross or microscopic, associated infection.
- TCC: see below.

Bladder

- Calculus: sudden cessation of micturition, pain in perineum and tip of penis.
- TCC: characteristically painless, intermittent haematuria, history of work in rubber or dye industries.
- Acute cystitis: suprapubic pain, dysuria, frequency and bacteriuria.
- Interstitial cystitis (rare): may be autoimmune, drug or radiation induced, frequency and dysuria common.
- Schistosomiasis (very rare): history of foreign travel, especially North Africa.

Prostate

- BPH: painless haematuria, associated obstructive symptoms, recurrent UTI.
- Carcinoma (rare).

Urethra

- Trauma: blood at meatus, history of direct blow to perineum, acute retention.
- Calculus (rare).
- Urethritis (rare).

26 Scrotal swellings

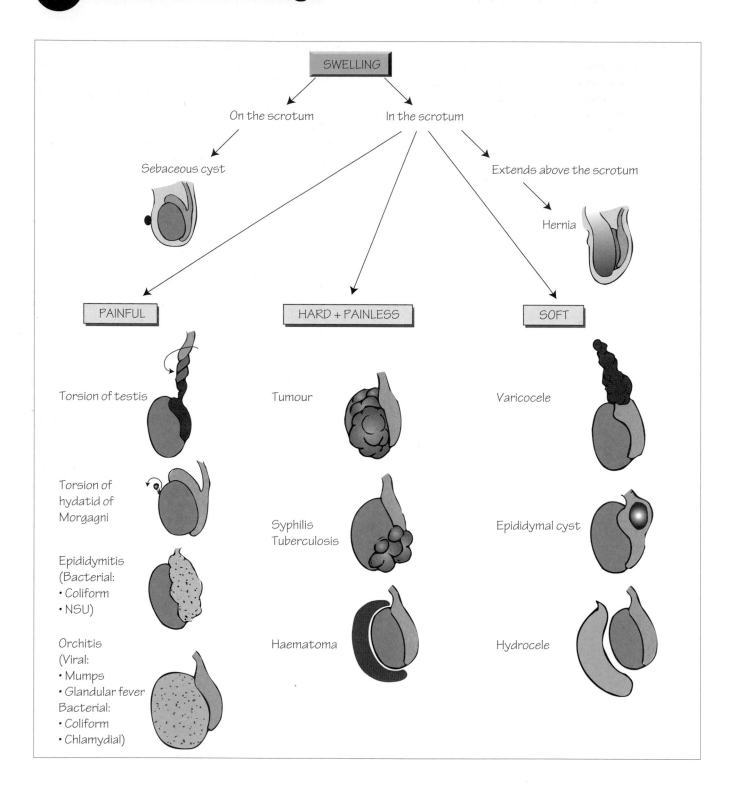

Definition

Any swelling in or on the scrotum or its contents.

> ## Key points
>
> • Always evaluate scrotal swellings for extension to the groin. If present they are almost always inguinoscrotal hernias.
> • Torsion is most common in adolescence and in the early twenties. Whenever the diagnosis is suspected, urgent assessment and usually surgery are required.
> • Young adult men: tumours, trauma and acute infections are common.
> • Older men: hydrocele and hernia are common.

Differential diagnosis

The causes and features are listed below.

Scrotum

• Sebaceous cyst: attached to the skin, just fluctuant, does not transilluminate.
• Infantile scrotal oedema: acute idiopathic scrotal swelling, hot, tender, bright red, testicle less tender than in torsion, most common in young boys.

Testis

Painful conditions

• Orchitis: confined to testis, young men (mumps, brucellosis)
• Epididymo-orchitis: painful and swollen, epididymis more than testis, associated erythema of scrotum, fever and pyuria, unusual below the age of 25 years, pain relieved by elevating the testis. May be related to sexually transmitted disease.
• Torsion of the testis: rapid onset, pubertal males, often high investment of tunica vaginalis on the cord—'bellclapper testis', testis may lie high and transversely in the scrotum, 'knot' in the cord may be felt.
• Torsion of appendix testis (hydatid of Morgagni): mimics full torsion, early signs are a lump at the upper pole of the testis and a blue spot on transillumination, later the whole testis becomes swollen, may require explorative surgery to exclude full torsion.

Hard conditions

• Testicular tumour: painless swelling, younger adult men (20–50 years), may have lax secondary hydrocele, associated abdominal lymphadenopathy.
• Haematocele: firm, does not transilluminate, testis cannot usually be felt, history of trauma.
• Syphilitic gummata—firm, rubbery, usually associated with other features of secondary syphilis. TB—uncommon, usually associated with miliary disease.

Soft conditions

• Hydrocele: soft, fluctuant, transilluminates brilliantly, testis may be difficult to feel, new onset or rapidly recurrent hydrocele suggests an underlying testicular cause.
• Epididymal cyst: separate and behind the testis, transilluminates well, may be quite large.
• Varicocele: a collection of dilated and tortuous veins in the spermatic cord—'bag of worms' on examination, more common on the left, associated with a dragging sensation, occasional haematospermia.

> ## Key investigations
>
> • FBC: infection.
> • Ultrasound: painless, non-invasive imaging of testicle. Allows underlying pathology to be excluded in hydrocele. High sensitivity and specificity for tumours.
> • Doppler ultrasound: may confirm presence of blood flow where torsion is thought unlikely.
> • CT scan: staging for testicular tumours.
> • Surgery: may be the only way to confirm or exclude torsion in a high-risk group. Should not be delayed for any other investigation if required.

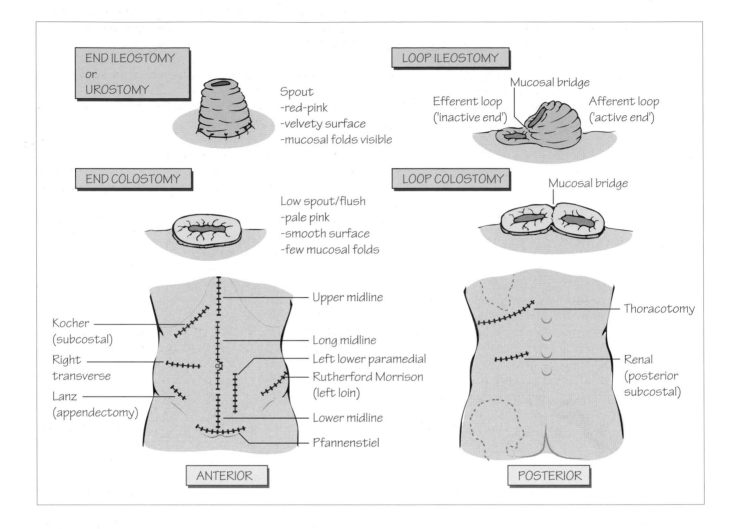

Definitions

A *stoma* is an opening from a hollow viscus connecting it to the skin surface. A *gastrostomy* is an opening into the stomach which is maintained by inserting a tube. An *ileostomy* is an opening in the small intestine. A *colostomy* is an opening in the large intestine. A *urostomy* is an external opening in the urinary tract. The most common form is a short length of ileum formed into a stoma and connected to the urinary tract (ureters) to act as a conduit for urine (ileal conduit). A *laparotomy* is any incision in the abdominal wall.

Key points

- Ileostomies and urostomies are usually spouted to reduce the risk of the output causing irritation of the surrounding skin.
- Colostomies are usually flush to the skin.
- Don't assume what type of stoma is present by its location.

Gastrostomies are almost always as a tube placed via the abdominal wall; placement is often by a percutaneous endoscopic technique (PEG) but may be via open surgery. They may be temporary or permanent.

Indications for common stomas

- Gastrostomy:
  temporary: inability to swallow (e.g. post CVA, during pharyngeal DXT)
  permanent: loss of swallowing (e.g. MS, MND)
- Ileostomy:
  end: following total proctocolectomy for ulcerative colitis
  loop: relief of distal obstruction; protection of distal anastomosis, diversion of the fecal stream (may be temporary)
- Colostomy:
  end: following abdominoperineal resection of rectum and anal canal for low rectal carcinoma—permanent. Following sigmoid colectomy for carcinoma or diverticulitis—may be temporary

loop: relief of distal obstruction; protection of distal anastomosis, diversion of the fecal stream (may be temporary)
• Ileal conduit: urinary diversion after cystectomy.

Complications of stomas
• Necrosis: acute early complication due to compromised blood supply—appears black or dark purple. Rx—re-operation to remake the stoma.
• Stenosis: narrowing of stoma or cutaneous orifice usually due to small skin defect or chronic ischaemia of stoma. Rx—dilatation by probe dilators or refashioning of stoma by surgery.
• Retraction: spout reduced/absent or stoma indrawn into abdominal wall, usually due to tension on the bowel used. Rx—convex stoma appliances, refashioning of stoma by surgery.
• Prolapse: excessive spout length, due to loose skin defect or chronic effect of bowel peristalsis. More common in loop stomas especially loop colostomies. Rx—stoma appliance change or refashioning of stoma.
• Herniation: presence of bowel in the subcutaneous tissues. Usually due to an oversized opening in the abdominal muscles wall. Most common long-term stoma complication. Often causes problems with stoma appliance adherence. Rx—repair hernia, resiting stoma.
• Peristomal dermatitis: due to contents spilling onto peristomal skin or trauma of appliance changes. Rx—better stoma care, change of appliance, topical anti-inflammatories.
• Fluid and electrolyte imbalances: usually only a problem in ileostomies (especially early after formation, if high in the small bowel or associated gastroenteritis). Caused by excessive wash-out of electrolyte rich fluid. Rx—control of high output (dietary modifications, use of anti-diarrhoeals, temporary use of isotonic oral fluids), intravenous fluid replacement if severe.

Features to recognize a stoma
Spout
• Fully spouted stomas are almost always formed from ileum. They may be an ileostomy or a urostomy.
• Spouted stomas with two lumens are always loop ileostomies. Look carefully to identify a second lumen as it may not be obvious.
• Flush stomas are usually colostomies.

Position
• Although ileostomies are often placed in the right lower abdomen and colostomies are placed in the left lower abdomen, location is never a good indication of what type of stoma is present.
Contents
• Stoma appliance contents: ileostomies usually produce semi-liquid green–brown output, colostomies usually produce solid/semi-solid faecal output. Beware—this is often unreliable in disease processes or soon after formation where the outputs may be similar. Urostomies drain clear fluid.

Siting and care of a stoma
• Electively formed stomas should be sited pre-operatively by the stoma specialist. Features to take into account are: abdominal size and shape, skin folds/creases (avoid), previous scars(avoid), level of the belt or dress line (place stomas above *or* below but not *on*), manual dexterity and visual impairment of patient.
• Stoma appliances are extremely varied: they may be one or two piece (separate bag and adherent flange), flat or convex, drainable or sealed, with or without odour filters.

Abdominal and thoracic incisions
• Vertical incisions are usually non-muscle splitting but traverse several or many myotomes/dermatomes.
• Transverse incisions are usually muscle splitting but are placed to lie in one or two myotomes/dermatomes.
• Midline vertical incisions can easily be extended to improve access to all parts of the abdomen but are often larger than transverse incisions placed over the area to be operated on.
• Midline vertical incisions tend to be used where the extent or type of surgery is large or uncertain.
• Transverse incisions tend to have a lower risk of wound hernia formation.
• Thoracotomy incisions are placed between ribs and are muscle splitting.
• Thoracotomy incisions may involve division or disarticulation of the rib above or below the incision.

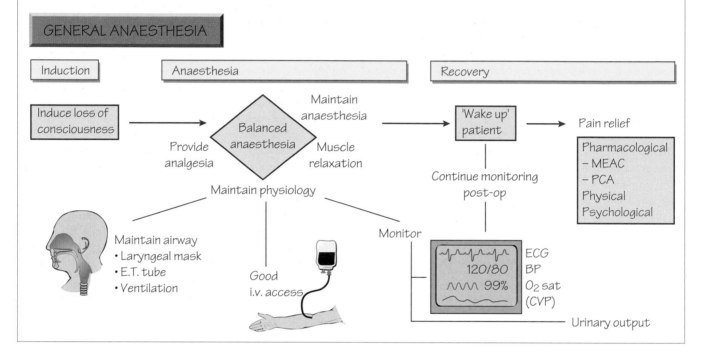

Definitions

Anaesthesia ($\alpha\nu\alpha\iota\sigma\theta\epsilon\sigma\iota\alpha$ = without perception): 1. a partial or complete loss of all forms of sensation caused by pathology in the nervous system, 2. a technique using drugs (inhalational, intravenous or local) that renders the whole or part of the organism insensible for variable periods of time. *Analgesia*: the loss of pain sensation. *Hypnotic agent*: a sleep-inducing drug. *Muscle relaxant*: a drug that reduces muscle tension by affecting the nerves that supply the muscles or the myoneuronal junction (e.g curare, succinylcholine). *Sedation*: the production of a calm and restful state by the administration of a drug.

Pre-operative assessment

Prior to an operation the anaesthetist will assess the patient and devise a plan for anaesthesia based on the following:

- The condition of the patient (ASA classification) determined by:
  history
  physical examination
  selective investigations
- The complexity of the surgery to be performed.
- The urgency of the procedure (emergency or elective).

Class	ASA pre-operative physical status classification
Class I	Fit and healthy
Class II	Mild systemic disease
Class III	Severe systemic disease that is not incapacitating
Class IV	Incapacitating systemic disease that is constantly life-threatening
Class V	Moribund—not expected to survive >24 hours without surgery

ASA = American Society of Anesthesiologists

General anaesthesia
Aims and technique

- To induce a loss of consciousness using hypnotic drugs which may administered intravenously (e.g. propofol) or by inhalation (e.g. sevoflurane).
- To provide adequate operating conditions for the duration of the surgical procedure using *balanced anaesthesia*, i.e. a combination of hypnotic drugs to maintain anaesthesia (e.g. propofol, sevoflurane), analgesics for pain (e.g. opiates, NSAIDs) and, if indicated, muscle relaxants (e.g. suxamethonium, tubocurarine) or regional anaesthesia.
- To maintain essential physiological function by:
  providing a clear airway (laryngeal mask airway or tracheal tube ± IPPV)
  maintaining good oxygenation (inspired O_2 concentration should be 30%)
  maintaining good vascular access (large-bore IV cannula ± central venous catheter ± arterial cannula)
  monitoring vital functions:
    - pulse oximetry (functional arterial O_2 saturation in %)
    - capnography (expired respiratory gas CO_2 level)
    - arterial blood pressure: non-invasive (sphigmomanometer) or invasive (arterial cannula) techniques
    - temperature
    - ECG
    - ± hourly urinary output, CVP
    - rarely: pulmonary arterial pressure, pulmonary capillary wedge pressure and cardiac output measure via a Swan–Ganz catheter or trans-oesophageal echocardiography.
- To awaken the patient safely at the end of the procedure.

Anaesthesia—regional

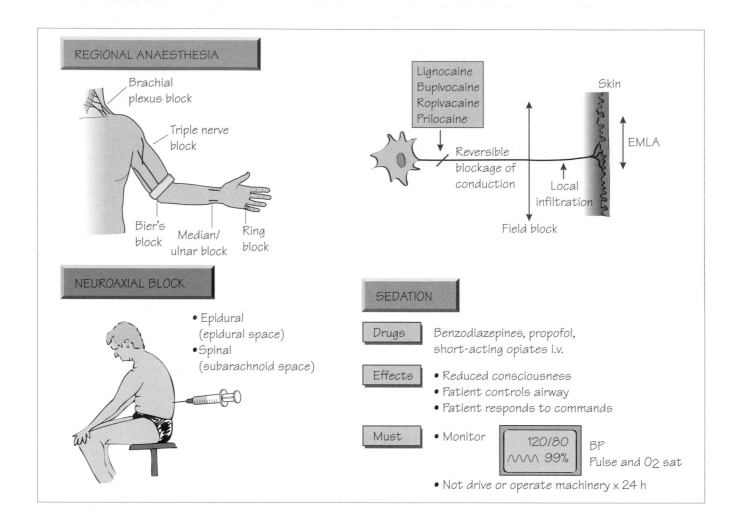

REGIONAL ANAESTHESIA

Brachial plexus block

Triple nerve block

Bier's block

Median/ulnar block

Ring block

Lignocaine
Bupivocaine
Ropivacaine
Prilocaine

Reversible blockage of conduction

Skin

EMLA

Local infiltration

Field block

NEUROAXIAL BLOCK

- Epidural (epidural space)
- Spinal (subarachnoid space)

SEDATION

Drugs — Benzodiazepines, propofol, short-acting opiates i.v.

Effects
- Reduced consciousness
- Patient controls airway
- Patient responds to commands

Must
- Monitor

120/80
99%

BP
Pulse and O₂ sat

- Not drive or operate machinery x 24 h

Regional anaesthesia

Aims and technique

- To render an area of the body completely insensitive to pain.
- LA agents prevent pain by causing a reversible block of conduction along nerve axons. Addition of a vasoconstrictor (e.g. adrenaline) reduces systemic absorption allowing more LA to be given and prolonging its duration of action.

	Dose, mg/kg (+ adrenaline)	Possible systemic toxicity of local anaesthetic agents
Lidocaine	3 (7)	CNS—drowsiness, confusion, visual disturbance,
Bupivacaine	2 (2)	headache, nausea, vomiting, convulsions
Ropivacaine	2 (2)	RS—respiratory arrest
Prilocaine	4 (7)	CVS—altered BP, arrhythmias, cardiac arrest

Regional anaesthetic techniques

- Topical administration of local anaesthetic (LA is placed on the skin, e.g. EMLA© cream prior to venepuncture).
- Local infiltration of LA (subcutaneous infiltration around the immediate surrounding area, e.g. used for excision of skin lesions).
- Field block (subcutaneous infiltration of LA around an operative field to render the whole operative field anaesthetic, e.g. used for inguinal hernia repair).
- Local blocks of specific peripheral nerves (± ultrasound guidance) (e.g. sciatic nerve block, ring block of fingers/toes, intercostals nerve block).
- Local blocks of specific plexuses (± ultrasound guidance) (e.g. brachial plexus block for upper limb surgery, coeliac plexus block for cancer pain).
- Intravenous blocks (e.g. Bier's block of the upper limb—a short-acting LA is injected via a cannula into an exsanguinated arm to which a tourniquet has been applied).

- Neuroaxial block:
  epidural anaesthesia: local anaesthetic is injected as a bolus or via a small catheter into the epidural space. It can be used as the sole anaesthetic for surgery below the waistline, especially useful in obstetrics, or as an adjunct to general anaesthesia.
  spinal anaesthesia: local anaesthetic is injected into the CSF in the subarachnoid space. The extent and duration of anaesthesia depend on the position of the patient, the specific gravity of the LA and the level of injection (usually lumbar spine level).

Sedation

Many minimally invasive procedures (e.g. colonoscopy) are performed under sedation only. Sedation is induced by administrating a drug or combination of drugs (e.g. benzodiazepines [midazolam], propofol ± short-acting opioids [pethidine, fentanyl]). During sedation the patient:

- has a reduced level of consciousness
- is free from anxiety
- is able to protect the airway
- is able to respond to verbal commands
- must be monitored (vital signs, pulse oximeter, ECG, level of consciousness)
- may be given an antagonist (naloxone, flumazenil) if oversedated (e.g. signs of respiratory depression).

After sedation the patient must be monitored until fully alert and must not drive or operate machinery for 24 hours.

Postoperative pain control

Pain is a complex symptom with physiological (*nociception* = neural detection of pain) and psychological (*anxiety, depression*) aspects. With modern analgesic techniques, postoperative pain should not be considered an inevitable consequence of surgery. *Neuopathic* pain is caused by damage to the nerve pathways.

Methods of analgesia:
- Pharmacological: drugs must achieve MEAC and may be administered:

oral	IV infusion
rectal	IV bolus
transdermal	IV patient controlled
subcutaneous	epidural
intramuscular	nerve blocks
(inhalational	Entonox – 50:50 oxygen:nitrous oxide)

- Physical:
  splinting, immobilization and traction
  physiotherapy
  TENS
- Psychological methods.

All hospitals should have an *acute pain team* to improve postoperative analgesia. PCA is a system whereby the patient can self-administer parenteral opioids to achieve pain relief. The system requires careful patient selection and monitoring but is a very effective method of pain relief.

Type of analgesic	Effects and mode of action	Side-effects
Non-opioid		
Paracetemol	• Analgesic and antipyretic Inhibits prostaglandin production centrally	Hepatic necrosis in large doses
NSAID Salicylates Acetic acids Propionic acids	• Analgesic, anti-inflammatory, antipyretic, antiplatelet Inhibit COX enzyme in peripheral tissue thus reducing prostaglandin induced inflammation and nociceptor stimulation. COX 2 inhibitors do not impair beneficial COX 1 effects (e.g. cytoprotection)	Gastric irritation and ulceration, altered haemostasis, CNS toxicity, renal impairment, asthma
Opioid Morphine Diamorphine Pethidine Fentanyl Codeine Tramadol	• Act on opioid receptors μ, κ, δ. Stimulation causes: μ–analgesia, RD, euphoria, dependence, N&V κ–spinal analgesia, sedation, miosiss δ–analgesia, RD euphoria, constipation	N&V, constipation, drowsiness, RD, tolerance, dependence
Adjuvant Antidepressants Anticonvulsants	• Analgesia (but not primary action of drug) Used mostly in chronic pain states	

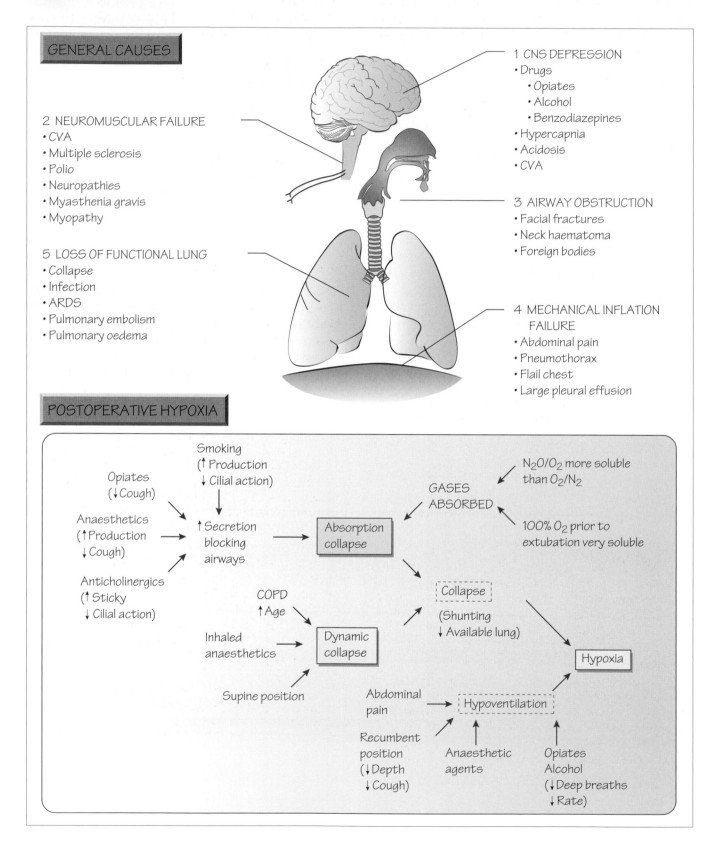

GENERAL CAUSES

1 CNS DEPRESSION
- Drugs
  - Opiates
  - Alcohol
  - Benzodiazepines
- Hypercapnia
- Acidosis
- CVA

2 NEUROMUSCULAR FAILURE
- CVA
- Multiple sclerosis
- Polio
- Neuropathies
- Myasthenia gravis
- Myopathy

3 AIRWAY OBSTRUCTION
- Facial fractures
- Neck haematoma
- Foreign bodies

5 LOSS OF FUNCTIONAL LUNG
- Collapse
- Infection
- ARDS
- Pulmonary embolism
- Pulmonary oedema

4 MECHANICAL INFLATION FAILURE
- Abdominal pain
- Pneumothorax
- Flail chest
- Large pleural effusion

POSTOPERATIVE HYPOXIA

Opiates ($\downarrow$Cough)

Smoking ($\uparrow$Production $\downarrow$Cilial action)

Anaesthetics ($\uparrow$Production $\downarrow$Cough)

$\uparrow$Secretion blocking airways

Anticholinergics ($\uparrow$Sticky $\downarrow$Cilial action)

Absorption collapse

N_2O/O_2 more soluble than O_2/N_2

GASES ABSORBED

100% O_2 prior to extubation very soluble

COPD $\uparrow$Age

Collapse (Shunting $\downarrow$Available lung)

Inhaled anaesthetics

Dynamic collapse

Hypoxia

Supine position

Abdominal pain

Hypoventilation

Recumbent position ($\downarrow$Depth $\downarrow$Cough)

Anaesthetic agents

Opiates Alcohol ($\downarrow$Deep breaths $\downarrow$Rate)

 Surgery at a Glance, 4e. By P. Grace and N.R. Borley. Published 2009 by Blackwell Publishing. ISBN 978-1-4051-8325-3.

Definitions

Hypoxia is defined as a lack of O_2 (usually meaning lack of O_2 delivery to tissues or cells). *Hypoxaemia* is a lack of O_2 in arterial blood. *Hypoventilation* is inadequate breathing leading to an increase of CO_2 (*hypercapnia*) and hypoxaemia. *Apnoea* means cessation of breathing in expiration.

Classification of hypoxia

• Hypoxic hypoxia: reduced O_2 entering the blood.
• Hypaemic/anaemic hypoxia: reduced capacity of blood to carry O_2.
• Stagnant hypoxia: poor oxygenation due to poor circulation.
• Histotoxic hypoxia: inability of cells to use O_2.

Common causes
Postoperative causes (usually hypoxic hypoxia)

• CNS depression, e.g. post-anaesthesia.
• Airway obstruction, e.g. aspiration of blood or vomit, laryngeal oedema.
• Poor ventilation, e.g. abdominal pain, mechanical disruption to ventilation.
• Loss of functioning lung, e.g. V/Q mismatch (pulmonary embolism, pneumothorax, collapse/consolidation).

General causes

• Central respiratory drive depression, e.g. opiates, benzodiazepines, CVA, head injury, encephalitis.
• Airway obstruction, e.g. facial fractures, aspiration of blood or vomit, thyroid disease or head and neck malignancy.
• Neuromuscular disorders (MS, myasthenia gravis).
• Obesity hypoventilation syndrome.
• Chest wall deformities.
• COPD.
• Shock.
• Carboxyhaemoglobinaemia, methaemoglobinaemia.

Key points

• 80% of patients following upper abdominal surgery are hypoxic during the first 48 hours postoperatively. Have a high index of suspicion and treat prophylactically.
• Adequate analgesia is more important than the sedative effects of opiates—ensure good analgesia in all postoperative patients.
• Ensure the dynamics of respiration are adequate—upright position, abdominal support, humidified O_2.
• Acutely confused (elderly) patients on a surgical ward are hypoxic until proven otherwise.
• Pulse oximetry saturations <85% equate to an arterial Po_2 <8 kPa and are unreliable in patients with poor peripheral perfusion.

Analgesia in postoperative patients

• Opiates: powerful, highly effective if given by correct route (e.g. PCA) but antitussive, sedative only in overdose.
• Epidural: excellent for upper abdominal/thoracic surgery, can cause hypotension by relative hypovolaemia.

Clinical features
In the unconscious patient

• Central cyanosis.
• Abnormal respirations.
• Hypotension.

In the conscious patient

• Central cyanosis.
• Anxiety, restlessness and confusion.
• Tachypnoea.
• Tachycardia, dysrhythmias (AF) and hypotension.

Key investigations

• Pulse oximetry saturations: monitors the percentage of haemoglobin that is saturated with O_2—gives a guide to arterial oxygenation, Very useful for patient monitoring.
• Arterial blood gases (Pco_2 Po_2 pH base excess): respiratory acidosis, metabolic acidosis later.
• Chest X-ray: ?collapse/pneumothorax/consolidation.
• ECG: AF.

Essential management

Airway control.
• Triple airway manoeuvre (mouth opening, head extension and jaw thrust), suction secretions, clear oropharynx.
• Consider endotracheal intubation in CNS depression/exhausted patients (rising Pco_2), neuromuscular failure.
• Consider surgical airway (cricothyroidotomy/minitracheostomy) in facial trauma, upper airway obstruction.
Breathing
• Position patient—upright.
• Adequate analgesia.
• Supplemental O_2—mask/bag/ventilation.
• Support respiratory physiology—physiotherapy, humidified gases, encouraging coughing, bronchodilators.
Circulatory support.
• Maintain cardiac output.
• Ensure adequate fluid resuscitation.
Determine and treat the cause.

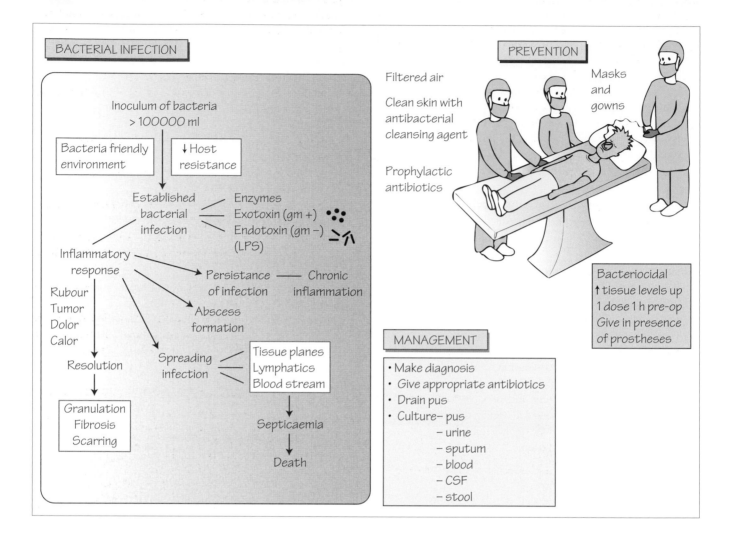

Definitions

Infection is the process whereby organisms (e.g. bacteria, viruses, fungi) capable of causing disease gain access and cause injury or damage to the body or its tissues. *Pus* is a yellow–green, foul-smelling, viscous fluid containing dead leucocytes, bacteria, tissue and protein. An *abscess* is localized collection of pus, usually surrounded by an intense inflammatory reaction. *Cellulitis* is a spreading infection of subcutaneous tissue.

Pathophysiology of bacterial infection

Establishing a bacterial infection requires:
• An inoculum of bacteria, (usually 100 000 organisms/mL exudate, or gram of tissue, or mm^2 surface area).
• A bacteria-friendly environment (water, electrolytes, carbohydrate, protein digests, blood).
• Diminished host resistance to infection (impaired physical barriers, reduced biochemical/humoral response, reduced cellular response).

Bacterial secretions

Bacteria cause some of their ill effects by releasing compounds:
• Enzymes (e.g. haemolysin, streptokinase, hyaluronidase).
• Exotoxin (released from intact bacteria, mostly Gram-positive, e.g. tetanus, diphtheria).
• Endotoxin (LPS released from cell wall on death of bacterium).

Natural history of infection

• Inflammatory response is established (rubor/redness, tumor/swelling, dolor/pain, calor/heat).
• Resolution: inflammatory reaction settles and infection disappears.
• Spreading infection:
  direct to adjacent tissues
  along tissue planes
  via lymphatic system (lymphangitis)
  via blood stream (bacteraemia)
• Abscess formation: localized collection of pus.

- Organization: granulation tissue, fibrosis, scarring.
- Chronic infection: persistence of organism in the tissues elicits a chronic inflammatory response.

> **Koch's postulates** for establishing a micro-organism as the cause of a disease.
>
>   The causative organism:
> - is present in all patients with the disease.
> - must be isolated from lesions in pure culture.
> - must reproduce the disease in susceptible animals.
> - must be re-isolated from lesions in the experimentally infected animals.

Management of surgical infection
Preventive measures
- Short operations.
- Skin cleansing with antibacterial chemicals and detergents (patient's, surgeons' and nurses' skin).
- Filtering of air in operating theatre.
- Occlusive surgical masks and gowns.
- Prophylactic antibiotics:
  should be bacteriocidal
  should have high tissue levels at time of contamination
  one pre-operative dose given 1 hour prior to surgery should suffice unless operation is heavily contaminated or dirty or the patient is immunocompromised.
  specific antibiotics should be given to patients with implanted prosthetic materials, e.g. heart valves, vascular grafts, joint prostheses.

Management of established infection
Diagnosis made by culture of appropriate specimens (pus, urine, sputum, blood, CSF, stool).
   Antibiotics:
- Prescribe on basis of culture results and 'most likely organism' while waiting for results.
- Certain antibiotics are reserved for serious infections—use the hospital policy wherever possible.
- Therapeutic monitoring of drug levels may be required, e.g. aminoglycosides.
- Synergistic combinations may be required in some infections, e.g. aminoglycoside, cephalosporin and metronidazole for faecal peritonitis.
- In serious, atypical or unresponsive infections seek advice from clinical microbiologist.
- Barrier nursing and isolation of patients with MRSA or VRE.
Drainage—surgical or radiological—is the most important treatment modality for an abscess or collections of infected fluid.

Wound classification	Definition	Example	Incidence of wound infection (%)
Clean	No contamination from GI, GU or RT	Thyroidectomy, elective hernia repair	1–5
Clean contaminated	Minimal contamination from GI, GU or RT	Cholecystectomy, TURP, pneumonectomy	7–10
Contaminated	Significantcontamination from GI, GU or RT	Elective colon surgery, inflamed appendicitis	15–20
Dirty	Infection present	Bowel perforation, perforated appendicitis, infected amputation	30–40

Surgical infection—specific

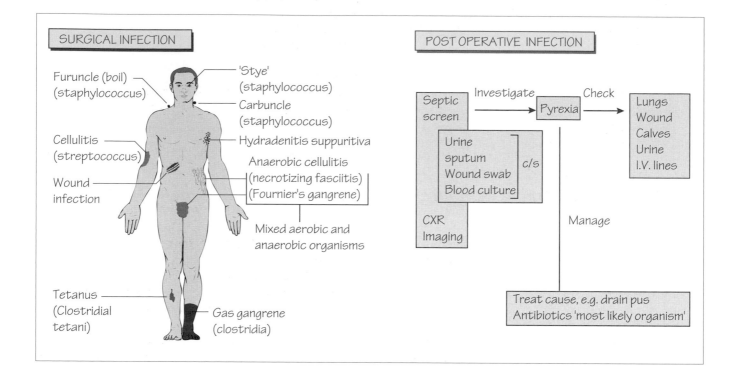

Specific surgical infections
Cellulitis
• Acute pyogenic cellulitis (*Streptococcus pyogenes*). Erysipelas (face) is most virulent form.
• Anaerobic cellulitis. Combination of aerobic (e.g. β-haemolytic streptococci) and anaerobic organisms (e.g. *Bacteroides*). Two forms clinically:
   progressive bacterial syergistic gangrene (including Fournier's gangrene)
   necrotizing fasciitis
   Treatment involves resuscitation, antibiotics (e.g. penicillin, metronidazole, gentamycin) and wide surgical débridement.
• Staphylococcal infections (*Staphlococcus aureus*, *Staph. epidermis*):
   furuncle (a boil)—skin abscess involving hair follicle
   stye—infection of eyelash follicle
   carabuncle—subcutaneous necrosis with network of small abscesses
   sycosis barbae—infection of shaving area caused by infected razor
• Hydradenitis suppuritiva—infection of apocrine glands in skin (axilla, groin).

Tetanus
• Clostridial infection caused by *Clostridium tetani*.
• Penetrating dirty wounds.
• Most symptoms caused by exotoxin which is absorbed by motor nerve endings and migrates to anterior horn cells:
   spastic contractions and trismus (lockjaw)

spasm of facial muscles (risus sardonicus)
rigidity and extensor convulsions (opisthotonos)

Standard tetanus prophylaxis in the UK	Tetanus toxoid is given during first year of life as part of triple vaccine. Booster at 5 years and end of schooling
Presentation with potentially contaminated wound + previous full immunization	Booster dose of tetanus toxoid given
Presentation with potentially contaminated wound – previous immunization	Passive immunization with human antitetanus immunoglobin Full course of active immunization commenced

Gas gangrene
• Clostridial infection caused by *C. perfringens* (85%), *C. septicum* (10%), *C. novyi* (5%).
• Contamination of necrotic wounds with soil containing *Clostridia*.
• Spreading gangrene of muscles with crepitus from gas formation, toxaemia and shock.
• Rx—resuscitation, complete débridement and excision of *all* infected tissue (may require several operations).

Postoperative infections
Pyrexia is a common sign of infection. A mildly raised temperature is normal in the early postoperative period indicating response to major surgery. If pyrexia develops:

<table>
<tr><td>

Note:
- Time of onset (first 24 hours usually atelectasis)
- Degree and type:
  (low persistent = low grade infectivity or inflammatory process, Intermittent = abscess ± rigors or haemodynamic change (bacteraemia/septicaemia)

Do:
- Septic screen:
  urine specimen
  sputum sample
  swabs of wounds or cannulae
  blood cultures
- Chest X-ray (± other imaging as indicated, e.g. abdominal U/S or CT scan if peritonitis present)

</td><td>

Check:
- Lungs (atelectasis/pneumonia)
- Wound (infection)
- Calves (DVT)
- Urine (infection)
- IV or central lines

Give:
Antibiotics on basis of 'most likely organism' (Refine treatment when septic screen results available)

Treat:
Cause as appropriate (e.g. remove infected cannula, drain abscess surgically or radiologically, give chest physiotherapy respiratory support, deal with anastomotic dehiscence, etc.)

</td></tr>
</table>

Wound infections
- Incidence depends on wound classification (see above).
- Mild may settle with antibiotics but most need wound to be opened and drained.

Intra-abdominal infections
- Generalized peritonitis—pain, rigidity, absence of bowel sounds.
- Depends on cause—typically: *E. coli*, *Klebsiella*, *Proteus*, *Strep. faecalis*, *Bacteroides*.
- Rx—resuscitation, broad-spectrum antibiotics, laparotomy and deal with cause if appropriate.

Intra-abdominal abscess
- Intermittent pyrexia, localized tenderness ± evidence of bacteraemia/septicaemia.
- Diagnosis by U/S or CT scanning.
- Rx—resuscitation, broad-spectrum antibiotics, drainage: either radiologically guided or open surgical.

Respiratory infections
- Predisposing factors:
  pre-existing pulmonary disease
  smoking
  starvation and fluid restriction
  anaesthesia
  postoperative pain
- Prevention:
  pre-operative physiotherapy
  incentive spirometry
  stop smoking
- Treatment:
  physiotherapy and appropriate antibiotics
  good postoperative analgesia
  keep well hydrated

Urinary tract infections
- Often related to urinary catheter.
- Only catheterize when necessary.
- Use sterile technique and closed drainage.
- Treat with antibiotic on basis of urine culture.

Intravenous central line infection
- Prevention:
  use sterile technique when inserting line
  don't use line for giving IV drugs or taking blood samples, especially if used for parenteral nutrition
  use single bag parenteral nutrition given over 24 hours
  never add anything to the parenteral nutrition bag
- Diagnosis: suspect it with any fever in a patient with a central line.
- Treatment: remove the line if possible, send tip of catheter for culture, antibiotics (via the line if kept).

Pseudomembranous enterocolitis
- Caused by *Clostridium difficile*.
- Seen in patients who have been on antibiotics (especially cephalosporins).
- Presents with diarrhoea, abdominal discomfort, leucocytosis.
- Dx: clinically—*C. difficile* +ve with above clinical picture, pseudomembranous membrane in the colon at endoscopy.
- Rx: resuscitate, stop current antibiotics, oral vancomycin or metronidazole, very rarely life-saving colectomy.

Multidrug-resistant organisms
- Micro-organisms resistant to to one or more classes of antimicrobial drugs (e.g. MRSA, VRE and some Gram-negative bacilli).
- May arise in health facilities or *de novo* in the community (e.g. CA-MRSA).
- Cause same infections as other micro-organisms but potentially more serious because of antimicrobial resistance.
- Prevention and control:
  infection prevention: improved hand hygiene, contact precautions (isolate patient, use gloves and masks for all patients)
  accurate, prompt diagnosis—treatment: active MDRO surveillance cultures
  judicious use of antimicrobials: MDROs are usually susceptible to certain antibiotics which should be reserved
  prevention of transmission: enhanced environmental cleaning, identify patients with MDROs, decolonization of carriers (especially MRSA)

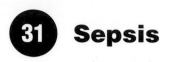

Sepsis

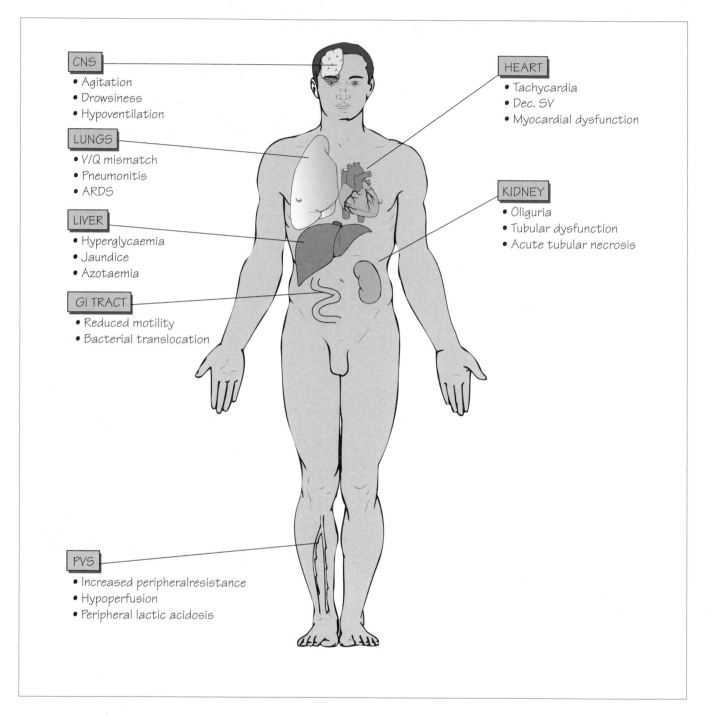

CNS
- Agitation
- Drowsiness
- Hypoventilation

LUNGS
- V/Q mismatch
- Pneumonitis
- ARDS

LIVER
- Hyperglycaemia
- Jaundice
- Azotaemia

GI TRACT
- Reduced motility
- Bacterial translocation

PVS
- Increased peripheralresistance
- Hypoperfusion
- Peripheral lactic acidosis

HEART
- Tachycardia
- Dec. SV
- Myocardial dysfunction

KIDNEY
- Oliguria
- Tubular dysfunction
- Acute tubular necrosis

Definitions

Sepsis is defined as the systemic response to the presence of various pathogenic organisms (bacteria—*bacteraemia*, viruses —*viraemia*, fungi—*fungaemia*) or their toxins (endotoxin— *lipopolysaccharide* or exotoxin—*tetanus/diphtheria toxin*) in the blood or tissues. Sepsis is a spectrum ranging from mild cellulitis to septic shock.

Septicaemia denotes the presence of large numbers of actively *dividing* bacteria in the blood stream, resulting in a systemic inflammatory response (SIRS, see Chapter 32) leading to organ dysfunction. *Pyaemia* is septicaemia caused by pus-forming bacteria (usually staphylococci) in the blood stream.

Severe sepsis denotes acute multiple organ dysfunction (MODS, see Chapter 32) secondary to infection.

 Surgery at a Glance, 4e. By P. Grace and N.R. Borley. Published 2009 by Blackwell Publishing. ISBN 978-1-4051-8325-3.

Septic shock is severe sepsis plus hypotension not reversed with fluid resuscitation (shock, see Chapter 33).

Epidemiology
The incidence of sepsis is 3/1000 worldwide and carries an overall mortality of 25%.

Risk factors
- Presence of an abscess or other source of infection (UTI, cholangitis, cellulitis, perforated viscus).
- Age: elderly and young most at risk.
- Immuno-compromised at risk:
  corticosteroids
  diabetes mellitus
  cancer chemotherapy
  burns
- Surgery or instrumentation can precipitate sepsis:
  urinary catheterization
  cannulization of biliary tree
  prostatic biopsy

Pathophysiology
The following may result from sepsis:
- Abnormal coagulation—cell apoptosis.
- Abnormal capillary permeability—increased neutrophil activity.
- Endothelial cell injury—poor glycaemic control.
- Elevated levels of tumour necrosis factor—reduced levels of steroid hormone.

Management		Supportive therapy	
Goal-directed early (first 6 hours) resuscitation	CVP 8–12 mmHg MAP ≥65 mmHg Urine output ≥0.5 mL/kg^{-1}/hour^{-1} Mixed venous O$_2$ Sat ≥65%	Mechanical ventilation of ALI/ARDS	Tidal vol. 6 mL/kg Use PEEP Elevate head of bed 30°
Diagnosis	Cultures before antibiotics Imaging to identify source of infection	Sedation, analgesia and neuromuscular blockade	Achieve sedation for mechanical ventilation Do not use neuromuscular blockade
Antibiotic therapy	Early (within 1 hour) IV antibiotics Empirical Rx against all likely pathogens Review regime daily	Glucose control	Give IV insulin to achieve blood glucose of 8.3 mmol/L
Source control	Seek specific anatomical source of infection amenable to control Treat source with least physiological insult, e.g. percutaneous vs. surgical drainage of an abscess	Renal replacement	Use continuous renal replacement therapy
Fluid therapy	Give either crystalloids or colloids to achieve CVP ≥8 mmHg Give fluid challenges, e.g. 1000 mL crystalloid over 30 min	Bicarbonate therapy	Do not use
Vasopressors	Noradrenaline or dopamine to maintain MAP of ≥65 mmHg Patients on vasopressors should have BP measured by an arterial line	DVT prophylaxis	Use heparin (low molecular weight in preference to unfractionated) ± mechanical prophylaxis (compression stockings or devices)
Inotropes	Dobutamine infusion in the presence of myocardial dysfunction		
Steroids	IV hydrocortisone in adults only when BP not responsive to adequate fluid resuscitation and vasopressors		
rhAPC	Only administer to adult patients with sepsis-induced multiple organ failure with a high risk of death (APACHE II ≥25)	Stress ulcer prophylaxis	Give H$_2$ blocker or PPI
Blood products	Maintain target Hb of 7.0–9.0 g/dL Do not use erythropoietin Only give FFP for coagulopathy in the presence of bleeding or prior to an invasive procedure Give platelets when ≤5000/mm^3 ≥50 000/mm^3 required for surgery	Consideration for limitation of support	Realistic outcomes should be discussed with patient and family Withdrawal of therapy may be in patient's best interest

Prognosis
Prognosis is related to the degree of sepsis but mortality is approximately 40% for established septic shock (see: www.survivingsepsis.org).

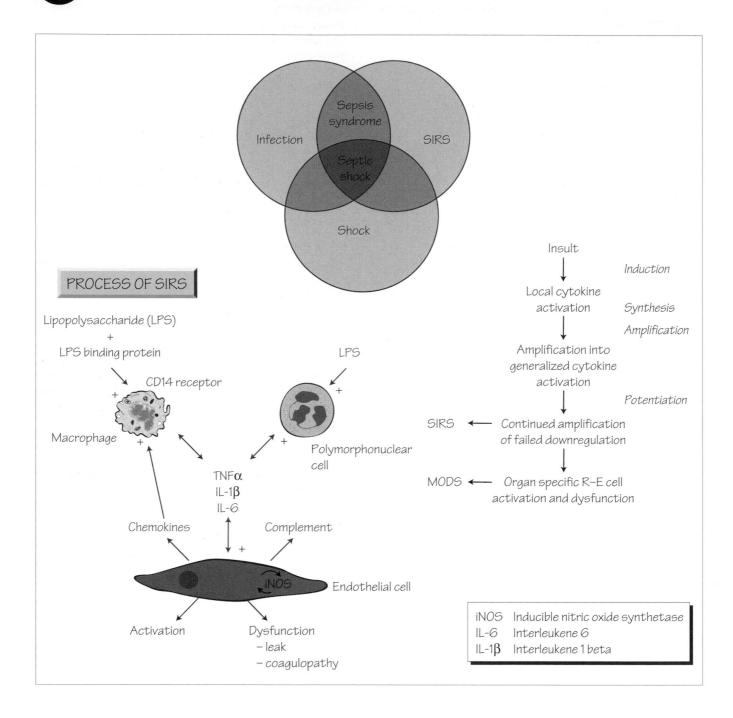

Definitions

Systemic inflammatory response syndrome (*SIRS*) is a systemic inflammatory response characterized by the presence of two or more of the following:

- Hyperthermia 38°C or hypothermia 36°C.
- Tachycardia > 90 beats/minute.
- Tachypnoea 20 beats/minute or Pa_{CO_2} 4.3 kPa.
- Neutrophilia $12 \times 10^{-9}/L^{-1}$ or neutropenia $4 \times 10^{-9}/L^{-1}$.
  Severe SIRS is as above plus one of the following:
- Organ dysfunction (e.g. jaundice, hypoglycaemia).
- Hypoperfusion (prolonged capillary refill time).
- Hypotension.

Sepsis syndrome is a state of SIRS with proven infection (SIRS + infection = sepsis). *Septic shock* is *sepsis* with systemic shock.

Multiple organ dysfunction syndrome (*MODS*) is a state of derangement of physiology such that organ function cannot maintain homeostasis. Usually involves two or more organ systems.

The common terminal pathways for organ damage and dysfunction are vasodilatation, capillary leak, intravascular coagulation and endothelial cell activation.

Key points

- SIRS is more common in surgical patients than is diagnosed.
- Early treatment of SIRS may reduce the risk of MODS developing.
- The role of treatment is to eliminate any causative factor and support the cardiovascular, respiratory and renal physiology until the patient can recover.
- Overall mortality is 7% for a diagnosis of SIRS, 14% for sepsis syndrome and 40% for established septic shock.

Common surgical causes

- Perforated viscus with peritonitis.
- Fulminant colitis.
- Multiple trauma.
- Acute pancreatitis.
- Burns.
- Massive blood transfusion.
- Aspiration pneumonia, PE.
- Ischaemia reperfusion injury.

Causation and treatments

TNFα

TNFα is both released by and activates macrophages and neutrophils. It is cytotoxic to endothelial cells and parenchymal cells of end organs. There is no clear evidence that anti-TNFα therapy is effective in SIRS.

Lipopolysaccharide

Released from Gram-negative bacterial cell walls, activates macrophages via attachment of LPS binding protein and activation of CD14 molecules on the cell surface. There is no proven value for anti-LPS antibody treatment.

Interleukines

IL-6 and IL-1β cause endothelial cell activation and damage. They promote complement and chemokines release. High-dose intravenous steroids have little role in established SIRS (probably because of multiple pathways of activation). Steroids for early SIRS are unproven.

Platelet-activating factor

Implicated particularly in acute pancreatitis, no proven role for anti-PAF antibody treatment.

Inducible nitric oxide synthetase

Synthesized by activated endothelial cells, iNOS activates endothelial cells and leucocytes, and is a potent negative ionotrope.

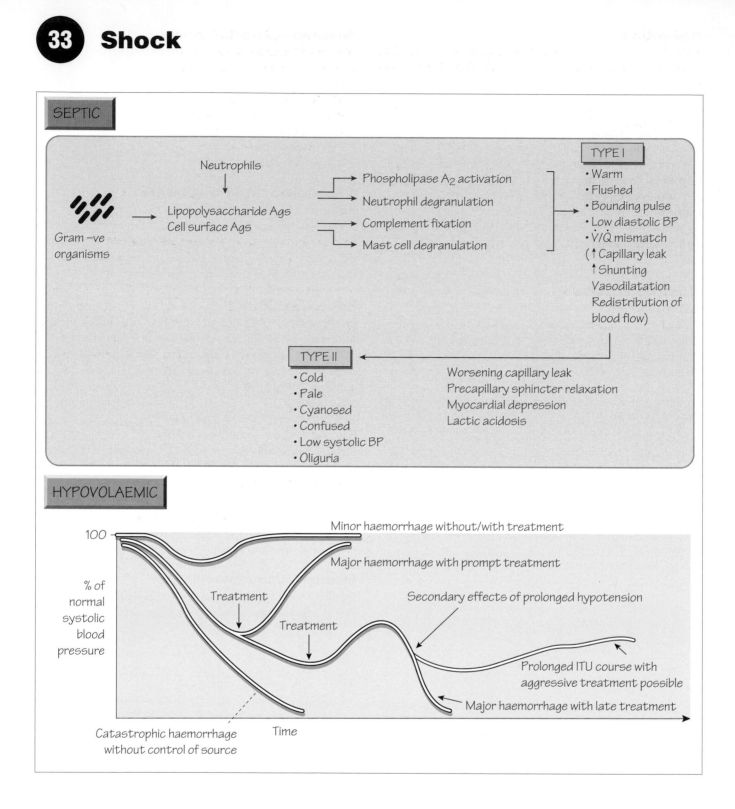

SEPTIC

Gram –ve organisms → Lipopolysaccharide Ags / Cell surface Ags

Neutrophils ↓

→ Phospholipase A$_2$ activation
→ Neutrophil degranulation
→ Complement fixation
→ Mast cell degranulation

TYPE I
• Warm
• Flushed
• Bounding pulse
• Low diastolic BP
• $\dot{V}/\dot{Q}$ mismatch
(↑Capillary leak
↑Shunting
Vasodilatation
Redistribution of
blood flow)

Worsening capillary leak
Precapillary sphincter relaxation
Myocardial depression
Lactic acidosis

TYPE II
• Cold
• Pale
• Cyanosed
• Confused
• Low systolic BP
• Oliguria

HYPOVOLAEMIC

% of normal systolic blood pressure

100

Minor haemorrhage without/with treatment
Major haemorrhage with prompt treatment
Treatment
Treatment
Secondary effects of prolonged hypotension
Prolonged ITU course with aggressive treatment possible
Major haemorrhage with late treatment
Catastrophic haemorrhage without control of source
Time

Definition

Shock is defined as a state of acute inadequate or inappropriate tissue perfusion resulting in generalized cellular hypoxia and dysfunction.

Key points

- Identify the cause early and begin treatment quickly.
- Shock in surgical patients is often overlooked—unwell, confused, restless patients may well be shocked.
- Unless a cardiogenic cause is obvious, treat shock with urgent fluid resuscitation.
- Worsening clinical status despite adequate volume replacement suggests the need for intensive care.

Common causes

Hypovolaemic

- Blood loss (ruptured abdominal aortic aneurysm, upper GI bleed, multiple fractures, etc.).
- Plasma loss (burns, pancreatitis).
- Extracellular fluid losses (vomiting, diarrhoea, intestinal fistula).

Cardiogenic

- Myocardial infarction.
- Dysrhythmias (AF, ventricular tachycardia, atrial flutter).
- Pulmonary embolus.
- Cardiac tamponade.
- Valvular heart disease.

Septic

Gram-negative or, less often, Gram-positive infections. Fungal —usually *Candida albicans*.

Anaphylactic/distributive

Release of vasoactive substances when a sensitized individual is exposed to the appropriate antigen.

Clinical features

Hypovolaemic and cardiogenic

- Pallor, coldness, sweating and restlessness.
- Tachycardia, weak pulse, low BP and oliguria.

Septic

- Initially warm, flushed skin and bounding pulse.
- Later confusion, low BP and low output picture.

Investigations and assessment

- Monitor pulse, BP, temperature, respiratory rate and urinary output.
- Establish good IV access and set up CVP line (± pulmonary artery catheterization with Swan–Ganz catheter—controversial). Intraosseous fluids can be used as a rescue technique when unable to establish IV access, especially in children.
- ECG, cardiac enzymes, echocardiography—transthoracic or transoesophageal—excellent in diagnosis and goal directed management of shock.
- Hb, Hct, U+E, creatinine.
- Group and crossmatch blood: haemorrhage.
- Blood cultures: sepsis.
- Arterial blood gases.

Complications

- SIRS (see Chapter 32) may ensue if shock not corrected.
- Acute renal failure (acute tubular necrosis).
- Hepatic failure.
- Stress ulceration.

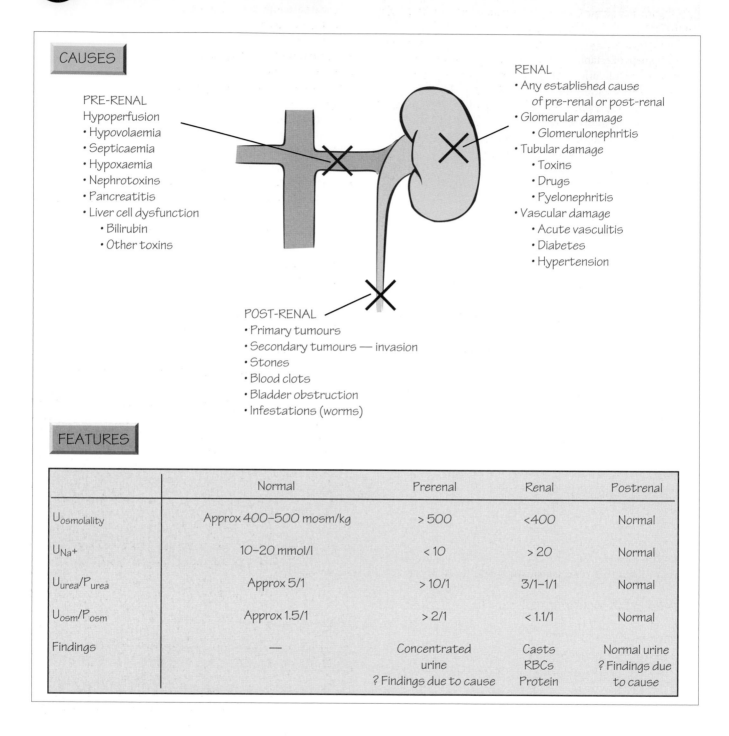

CAUSES

PRE-RENAL
Hypoperfusion
• Hypovolaemia
• Septicaemia
• Hypoxaemia
• Nephrotoxins
• Pancreatitis
• Liver cell dysfunction
  • Bilirubin
  • Other toxins

RENAL
• Any established cause
  of pre-renal or post-renal
• Glomerular damage
  • Glomerulonephritis
• Tubular damage
  • Toxins
  • Drugs
  • Pyelonephritis
• Vascular damage
  • Acute vasculitis
  • Diabetes
  • Hypertension

POST-RENAL
• Primary tumours
• Secondary tumours — invasion
• Stones
• Blood clots
• Bladder obstruction
• Infestations (worms)

FEATURES

	Normal	Prerenal	Renal	Postrenal
$U_{osmolality}$	Approx 400–500 mosm/kg	> 500	<400	Normal
U_{Na^+}	10–20 mmol/l	< 10	> 20	Normal
U_{urea}/P_{urea}	Approx 5/1	> 10/1	3/1–1/1	Normal
U_{osm}/P_{osm}	Approx 1.5/1	> 2/1	< 1.1/1	Normal
Findings	—	Concentrated urine ? Findings due to cause	Casts RBCs Protein	Normal urine ? Findings due to cause

Definitions

Acute renal failure (ARF) (also known as acute kidney injury (AKI)) is a sudden deterioration in renal filtration function such that neither kidney is capable of excreting body waste products (e.g. urea, creatinine, potassium) that accumulate in the blood. It may be fatal unless treated. *Anuria* means no urine is passed. *Oliguria* means that <0.5 mL/kg/hour is passed. *Acute tubular necrosis (ATN)* is damage to the renal tubular cells caused by ischaemia or nephrotoxins.

Common causes

Pre-renal failure (volume depletion and hypotension, structurally intact nephrons)

• Shock from any cause causing reduced renal perfusion (hypovolaemia, haemorrhage, burns, pancreatitis, sepsis, anaphylaxis, heart failure).
• Arteriolar vascoconstriction leading to ARF can occur with hypercalcaemia, radiocontrast agents and NSAIDs, ACE inhibitors, angiotensin receptor blockers and the hepatorenal syndrome.

Intrinsic renal failure (structural and functional damage to kidney)

• Vascular: renal ischaemia (ATN).
• Glomerular: acute glomerulonephritis.
• Tubular (ATN):
  ischaemic
  cytotoxic (*aminoglycosides*, amphotericin B, radiocontrast agents, methotrexate, myoglobin)
• Interstitial:
  drugs (penicillins, NSAIDs, allopurinol)
  infection (severe pyelonephritis)
• Systemic: hypertension, diabetes mellitus, myeloma.

Post-renal failure (obstruction to the passage of urine)

• Urinary tract obstruction.
• Ureteric (fibrosis, stone disease).
• Bladder neck (common) (benign prostatic hypertrophy, cancer of the prostate, neurogenic bladder).
• Urethra (stricture, phimosis).

Clinical features

Oliguric phase

(May last hours/days/weeks.)
• Oliguria: passage of <0.5 mL/kg/hour urine
• Uraemia: dyspnoea, confusion, drowsiness, coma.
• Nausea, vomiting, hiccoughs, diarrhoea.

• Anaemia, coagulopathy, GI haemorrhage.
• Fluid retention: hypervolaemia, hypertension.
• Hyperkalaemia: dysrrhythmias.
• Metabolic acidosis.

Polyuric (recovery) phase

(May last days/weeks.)
• Polyuria: hypovolaemia, hypotension.
• Hyponatraemia.
• Hypokalaemia.

Investigations

• Urinalysis (see opposite page).
• U+E (especially K^+) and creatinine.
• Arterial blood gases: metabolic acidosis (normal Po_2, low Pco_2, low pH, high base deficit).
• ECG/chest X-ray/renal ultrasound/renal biopsy.

Prognosis

In hospital mortality 40–50%, ICU 70–80%.

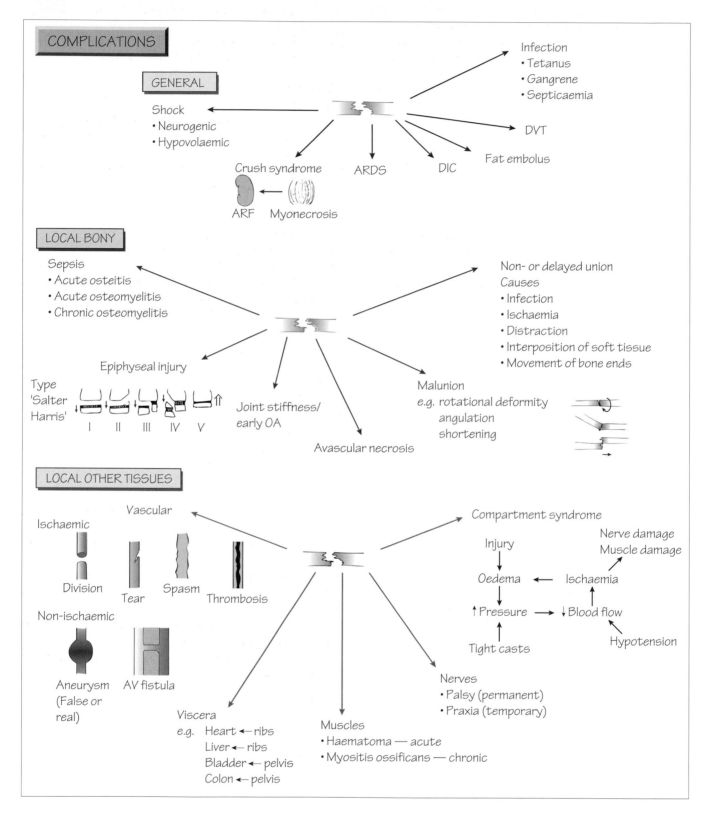

COMPLICATIONS

GENERAL

Infection
• Tetanus
• Gangrene
• Septicaemia

DVT

Fat embolus

Shock
• Neurogenic
• Hypovolaemic

Crush syndrome

ARDS

DIC

ARF   Myonecrosis

LOCAL BONY

Sepsis
• Acute osteitis
• Acute osteomyelitis
• Chronic osteomyelitis

Non- or delayed union
Causes
• Infection
• Ischaemia
• Distraction
• Interposition of soft tissue
• Movement of bone ends

Epiphyseal injury

Type 'Salter Harris'   I   II   III   IV   V

Joint stiffness/ early OA

Avascular necrosis

Malunion
e.g. rotational deformity
        angulation
        shortening

LOCAL OTHER TISSUES

Vascular

Ischaemic

Division   Tear   Spasm   Thrombosis

Non-ischaemic

Aneurysm (False or real)   AV fistula

Compartment syndrome

Injury

Oedema ← Ischaemia

↑Pressure → ↓Blood flow

Tight casts   Hypotension

Nerve damage
Muscle damage

Nerves
• Palsy (permanent)
• Praxia (temporary)

Viscera
e.g. Heart ← ribs
        Liver ← ribs
        Bladder ← pelvis
        Colon ← pelvis

Muscles
• Haematoma — acute
• Myositis ossificans — chronic

Definitions

A *fracture* is a break in the continuity of a bone. Fractures may be *transverse*, *oblique* or *spiral* in shape. In a *greenstick* fracture, only one side of the bone is fractured, the other simply bends (usually immature bones). A *comminuted* fracture is one in which there are more than two fragments of bone. In a *complicated* fracture, some other structure is also damaged (e.g. a nerve or blood vessel). In a *compound* fracture, there is a break in the overlying skin (or nearby viscera) with potential contamination of the bone ends. A *pathological* fracture is one through a bone weakened by disease, e.g. a metastasis.

Key points

- Always consider multiple injury in patients presenting with fractures.
- Compound fractures are a surgical emergency and require appropriate measures to prevent infection, including tetanus prevention.
- Always image the joints above and below a long bone fracture.

Common causes

Fractures occur when excessive force is applied to a normal bone or moderate force to a diseased bone, e.g. osteoporosis.

Clinical features

- Pain.
- Loss of function.
- Deformity, tenderness and swelling.
- Discoloration or bruising.
- (Crepitus—not to be elicited!)

Investigations

- Radiographs in two planes (look for lucencies and discontinuity in the cortex of the bone).
- Tomography, CT scan, MRI scan (rarely).
- Ultrasonography and radioisotope bone scanning. (Bone scan is particularly useful when radiographs/CT scanning are negative in clinically suspect fracture.)

Essential management

General

- Look for shock/haemorrhage and check ABC (see Chapter 37).
- Look for injury in other areas at risk (head and spine, ribs and pneumothorax, femoral and pelvic injury).

The fracture

Immediate

- Relieve pain (opiates IV, nerve blocks, splints, traction).
- Establish good IV access and send blood for group and crossmatch.
- Open (compound) fractures require débridement, antibiotics and tetanus prophylaxis.

Definitive

- Reduction (closed or open).
- Immobilization (casting, functional bracing, internal fixation, external fixation, traction).
- Rehabilitation (aim to restore the patient to pre-injury level of function with physiotherapy and occupational therapy).

Complications

Early

- Blood loss.
- Infection.
- Fat embolism.
- DVT and PE.
- Renal failure.
- Compartment syndrome.

Late

- Non-union (no sign of healing after 3–6 months, depending on fracture site)
- Delayed union (incomplete healing of a fracture at the expected time of healing).
- Malunion (bone fragments join in an unsatisfactory position).
- Growth arrest.
- Arthritis.
- Myositis ossificans (calcification within muscle especially in supracondylar humeral fracture).
- Post-traumatic sympathetic (reflex) dystrophy (Sudeck's atrophy).

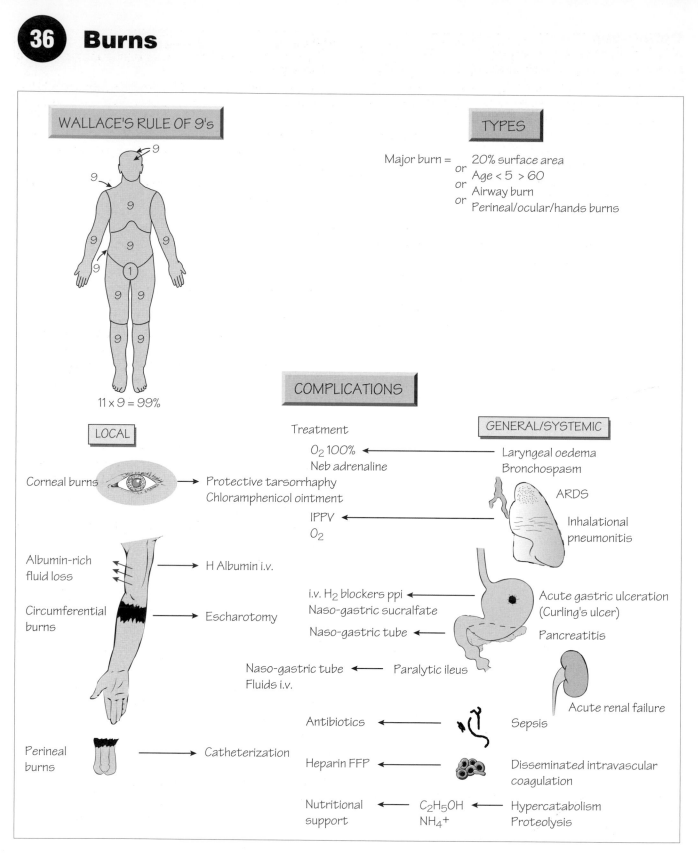

WALLACE'S RULE OF 9's

9
9
9
9 9 9
9 1
9 9
9 9

11 × 9 = 99%

TYPES

Major burn = or 20% surface area
or Age < 5 > 60
or Airway burn
or Perineal/ocular/hands burns

COMPLICATIONS

Treatment
O_2 100%
Neb adrenaline

IPPV
O_2

GENERAL/SYSTEMIC

Laryngeal oedema
Bronchospasm

ARDS

Inhalational pneumonitis

LOCAL

Corneal burns → Protective tarsorrhaphy
Chloramphenicol ointment

Albumin-rich fluid loss → H Albumin i.v.

Circumferential burns → Escharotomy

i.v. H_2 blockers ppi ← Acute gastric ulceration (Curling's ulcer)
Naso-gastric sucralfate

Naso-gastric tube ← Pancreatitis

Naso-gastric tube ← Paralytic ileus
Fluids i.v.

Acute renal failure

Antibiotics ← Sepsis

Perineal burns → Catheterization

Heparin FFP ← Disseminated intravascular coagulation

Nutritional support ← C_2H_5OH ← Hypercatabolism
NH_4^+ Proteolysis

Definitions

A *burn* is the response of the skin, mucous membranes and sub-cutaneous tissues to thermal injury. A *partial thickness* burn is a burn that either does not destroy the skin epithelium or destroys only part of it. (Partial thickness burns are subclassified into *superficial partial thickness* and *deep partial* thickness—may be difficult to distinguish between them). Partial thickness burns usually heal with conservative management. A *full thickness* burn destroys all sources of skin epithelial regrowth and may require excision and skin grafting if large.

Key points

- Start resuscitation immediately in major burns.
- Calculate fluid requirement from the time of the burn.
- Be sure to assess for vital area burns (airway/hands/face/perineum/circumferential).
- Assume that all burns in <5 years and >55 years are not superficial.
- Refer all major burns to a specialist burns centre.
- Remember tetanus prophylaxis.

Common causes

- Thermal injury from dry (flame, hot metal, sunburn) or moist (hot liquids or gases) heat sources.
- Electricity (deep burns at entry and exit sites, may cause cardiac arrest).
- Chemicals (usually industrial accidents with acid or alkali).
- Radiation (partial thickness initially, but may progress to chronic deeper injury).

Clinical features
General

Classification	Appearance	Sensation	Healing	Scarring
Superficial	Dry, red, blanches on pressure	Painful	3–6 days	None
Superficial partial	Blisters, moist, blanches on pressure	Painful	7–20 days	Unusual
Deep partial	Blisters, wet or waxy, no blanching on pressure	Pressure	>21 days	Severe
Full thickness	Waxy white to black, dry no blanching on pressure	None	Never	Very severe

Specific

- Evidence of smoke inhalation (soot in nose or sputum, burns in the mouth, hoarseness).
- Eye or eyelid burns (early ophthalmological opinion).
- Circumferential burns (will need escharotomy).
- Hands, feet, genitalia, joints (will need specialist care).

Investigations

- FBC.
- U+E.
- If inhalation suspected: chest X-ray, arterial blood gases, CO estimation.
- Blood group and crossmatch.
- ECG/cardiac enzymes with electrical burns.

Complications
Immediate

Compartment syndrome from circumferential burns (limb burns → limb ischaemia, thoracic burns → hypoxia from restrictive respiratory failure) (prevent by urgent escharotomy).

Early

- Hyperkalaemia (from cytolysis in large burns). Treat with insulin and dextrose.
- Acute renal failure (combination of hypovolaemia, sepsis, tissue toxins). Prevent by aggressive early resuscitation, ensuring high GFR with fluid loading and diuretics, treat sepsis.
- Infection (beware of *Streptococcus*). Treat established infection (10^6 organisms present in wound biopsy) with systemic antibiotics.
- Stress ulceration (Curling's ulcer) (prevent with antacid, H_2-blocker or PPI prophylaxis).

Late

Contractures.

Essential management
General

- Start resuscitation (ABC, see Chapter 37), set up good IV lines, give O_2).
- Assess size of burn (Wallace's rule of 9's)—in children the head is >9%, a child's palm = 1% of its total body surface area.
- Calculate fluid requirements from time of burn *not* time of admission.

Major burns (>10% burn in adult, >5% in child)

- Monitor pulse, BP, temperature, urinary output, give adequate analgesia IV, consider nasogastric tube, give tetanus prophylaxis.
- Give IV fluids according to Muir–Barclay formula:
  % burn × weight in kg/2 = one aliquot of fluid.
  Give six aliquots of fluid over first 36 h in 4, 4, 4, 6, 6, 12-hour sequence from time of burn. Colloid, albumin or plasma solutions are used.
- The burn wound is treated as for minor burns (see below).
- Consider referral to a burns centre.

Minor burns (<10% burn in adult, <5% in child)

- Treatment by exposure—débride wound and leave exposed in special clean environment.
- Treatment by dressings—cover with tulle gras impregnated with chlorhexidine or silver sulphadiazine under absorptive gauze dressings.
- Débridement of eschar and split skin grafting preferably in the first 5–10 days.

Criteria for referral to burns centre

- Partial thickness burn >10% total body surface area.
- Burns of face, hands, feet, genitalia, perineum, major joints.
- All full thickness burns.
- Electrical or chemical burns.
- Inhalation injury.
- Burns with concomitant major trauma or pre-existing medical conditions.
- Burned children.

Major trauma—basic principles

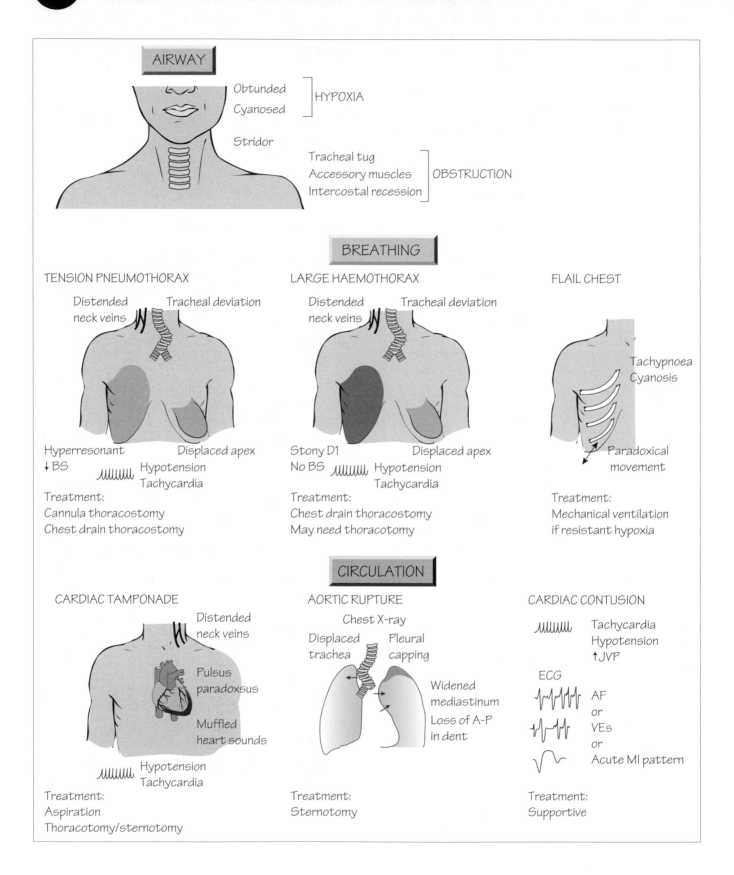

AIRWAY

Obtunded
Cyanosed
] HYPOXIA

Stridor

Tracheal tug
Accessory muscles] OBSTRUCTION
Intercostal recession

BREATHING

TENSION PNEUMOTHORAX

Distended neck veins   Tracheal deviation

Hyperresonant   Displaced apex
↓BS   Hypotension
Tachycardia

Treatment:
Cannula thoracostomy
Chest drain thoracostomy

LARGE HAEMOTHORAX

Distended neck veins   Tracheal deviation

Stony D1   Displaced apex
No BS   Hypotension
Tachycardia

Treatment:
Chest drain thoracostomy
May need thoracotomy

FLAIL CHEST

Tachypnoea
Cyanosis

Paradoxical movement

Treatment:
Mechanical ventilation
if resistant hypoxia

CIRCULATION

CARDIAC TAMPONADE

Distended neck veins

Pulsus paradoxsus

Muffled heart sounds

Hypotension
Tachycardia

Treatment:
Aspiration
Thoracotomy/sternotomy

AORTIC RUPTURE

Chest X-ray

Displaced trachea   Pleural capping

Widened mediastinum
Loss of A-P in dent

Treatment:
Sternotomy

CARDIAC CONTUSION

Tachycardia
Hypotension
↑JVP

ECG

AF
or
VEs
or
Acute MI pattern

Treatment:
Supportive

Definition

Major trauma (MT) can be defined as injury (or injuries) of organs of severity sufficient to present an immediate threat to life. MT often involves multiple injuries. The majority of patients who reach hospital alive following MT have potentially survivable injuries if detected and treated early.

Key points

- Treat all MT patients as having a potentially unstable cervical spine.
- Treat life-threatening injuries identified in the primary survey immediately upon discovery.
- Undiagnosed hypotension is due to occult haemorrhage unless proven otherwise.
- Commence rapid IV infusion immediately (warmed if possible).
- Emergency surgery may be part of the resuscitation of patients suffering from internal haemorrhage.

Principles of management

Management for MT is divided into two categories.
- **'First aid'**—'roadside' given by paramedics or on-site medical teams. Aims to maintain life during extraction and evacuation of patient.
- **Primary survey**—in hospital performed by accident and emergencyor trauma teams. Aims to identify and treat immediately life-threatening injuries to airways, respiratory and cardiovascular systems using **ABCDE** (see below). Important to: reasess repeatedly, treat life-threatening conditions as soon as diagnosed, leave penetrating wounds and implements for formal surgical exploration, stop external bleeding by direct pressure.
- **Secondary survey**—aim to document any other injuries, take history, examine patient from head to toe, document GCS, asses neck (clinical and radiology to include C7–T1) and perform major skeletal radiology.
- **Definitive treatment**—follows primary and secondary surveys and will depend on what injuries are present.

Patterns of injury

Some of the major injuries that may be encountered in the primary survey are shown opposite. Mechanisms of injury and patterns of injury may be associated, e.g.

Restrained RTA	Pedestrian collision
Cervical spine injury	Long bone fractures
Sternal fracture	Knee ligamentous injury
Cardiac contusion	Rib fractures
Liver laceration	Pneumothorax
	Facial fractures
	Head injury

Timing of death following trauma

- 1st peak: immediately at time of injury due to primary injury.
- 2nd peak: up to several hours post injury due to secondary injury, e.g. hypoxia, haemorrhage. Secondary injuries are frequently avoidable or treatable (e.g. chest drain for pneumothorax).
- 3rd peak: days or weeks post injury due to sepsis or multiple organ failure.

Essential management of trauma

Cervical spine
- Stabilize with in-line manual traction
  Lateral C spine/X-ray (must include C7–T1).
- Secure with hard collar, head supports and tape.
- Can only be 'cleared' by normal examination in a fully conscious patient or normal X-rays.

A Airway management (see opposite for major abnormalities)
- Clear obstructions by hand and lift chin (obtunded patients).
- Secure airway with oropharyngeal or nasopharyngeal airway (obtunded patients).
- Definitive airway (direct access to intratracheal oxygenation) indicated by:
  apnoea/(risk of) upper airway obstruction/(risk of) aspiration/need for mechanical ventilation
  orotracheal tube
  nasotracheal tube
- Surgical airway (cricothyroidotomy) indicated by: *maxillofacial injuries/laryngeal disruption/failure to intubate.*

B Breathing (see opposite for some major abnormalities)
- Administer supplemental O_2.
- Assess respiratory rate/air entry CXR (symmetry)/chest wall motion (symmetry)/tracheal position.
- Monitor with pulse oximetry and observations.

C Circulation (see opposite for some major abnormalities)
- Assess pulse rate and character/blood pressure/ apex beat/JVP/heart sounds/evidence of blood loss.
- Draw blood for crossmatch, FBC and U+E.

D Dysfunction of the CNS
- Assess GCS (see Chapter 38)/pupil reactivity/limb gross motor and sensory function where possible.

E Exposure of extremities
- Assess limbs for major long bone injuries and sites of major blood loss/pelvic x-ray.

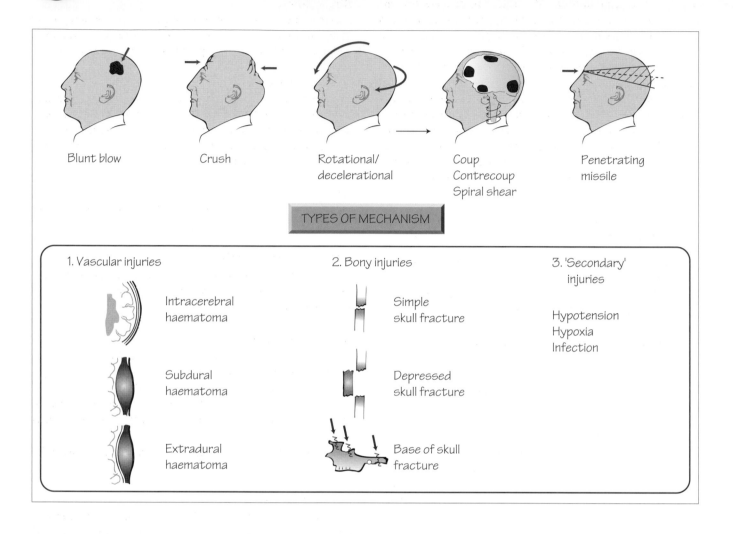

Blunt blow   Crush   Rotational/ decelerational   Coup Contrecoup Spiral shear   Penetrating missile

TYPES OF MECHANISM

1. Vascular injuries

Intracerebral haematoma

Subdural haematoma

Extradural haematoma

2. Bony injuries

Simple skull fracture

Depressed skull fracture

Base of skull fracture

3. 'Secondary' injuries

Hypotension
Hypoxia
Infection

Definitions

A *head injury* is the process whereby direct or decelerating trauma to the head results in skull and/or brain damage. *Primary brain injury* is the damage that occurs to the brain immediately as the result of the trauma. The degree of primary brain injury is directly related to the amount of force applied to the head. Prevention (e.g. helmets, airbags) is the only way to reduce primary injury.

Secondary brain injury is the damage that develops later as a result of complications. Secondary damage results from respiratory complications (*hypoxia, hypercarbia, airway obstruction*), hypovolaemic shock (head injury does not cause hypovolaemic shock—look for another cause), intracranial bleeding, cerebral oedema, epilepsy, infection and hydrocephalus. *Brain death* is defined as the absence of brain function.

Key points

- Prevention of secondary brain injury is the most important objective of head injury care.
- A full trauma survey (see Chapter 37) must be carried out on all patients with head injuries.
- The GCS provides a simple method of monitoring global CNS function over a period rather than a precise index of brain injury at any one time.
- 100% of those with severe head injury and 60% of moderate head injury will be permanently disabled.

Epidemiology

Head injury is very common. RTAs, falls, assaults and sports injuries are common causes. A million patients each year present to accident and emergency departments in the UK with head injury and about 5000 patients die each year following head injuries.

Pathophysiology
Closed head injury
Direct blow

May cause damage to the brain at the site of the blow (*coup injury*) or to the side opposite the blow when the brain moves within the skull and hits the opposite wall (*contrecoup injury*).

Rotation/deceleration

Neck flexion, extension or rotation results in the brain striking bony points within the skull (e.g. the wing of the sphenoid bone). Severe rotation also causes shear injuries within the white matter of the brain and brainstem, causing axonal injury and intracerebral petechial haemorrhages.

Crush

The brain is often remarkably spared direct injury unless severe (especially in children with elastic skulls).

Penetrating head injury

Missiles tend to cause loss of tissue with injury proportionate. Brain swelling—less of a problem due to the skull disruption automatically decompressing the brain.

Clinical features

- History of direct trauma to head or deceleration.
- Patient must be assessed fully for other injuries.
- Level of consciousness determined by GCS.
- Neurological assessment: brainstem tests: pupillary exam, ocular movements, corneal reflex, gag reflex; motor exam, sensory exam, reflex exam.
- Headache, nausea, vomiting, a falling pulse rate and rising BP indicate cerebral oedema.

Investigations

- Skull X-ray: AP, lateral and Towne's views. May be useful in penetrating head injury. Rarely used now to evaluate closed head injury. Plain radiographs are used to exclude cervical spine injury.
- CT/MRI scan: show contusions, haematomas, hydrocephalus, cerebral oedema. CT is diagnostic study of choice.

Glasgow Coma Scale.					
Eye opening		Voice response		Best motor response	
Spontaneous	4	Alert and orientated	5	Obeys commands	6
To voice	3	Confused	4	Localizes pain	5
To pain	2	Inappropriate	3	Flexes to pain	4
No eye opening	1	Incomprehensible	2	Abnormal flexion to pain	3
		No voice response	1	Extends to pain	2
				No response to pain	1
Fully conscious: GCS = 15; deep coma: GCS = 3.					

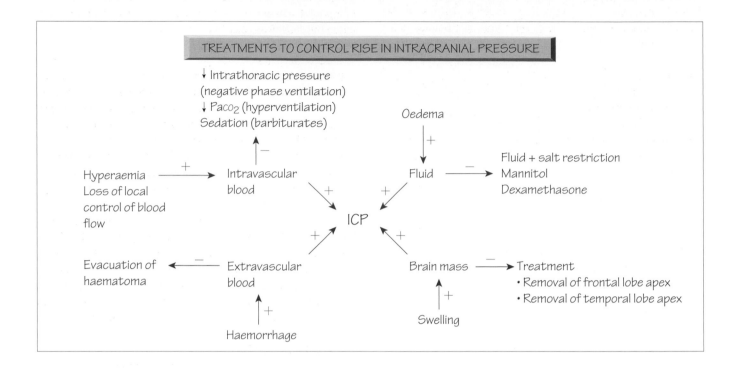

Essential management

Trivial head injury

The patient is conscious, may be history of period of LOC. Retrograde amnesia for events prior to head injury is significant.

Indications for CT scan

- LOC or amnesia.
- Neurological signs.
- CSF leakage.
- Suspected penetrating injury.
- Alcohol intoxication.
- Difficulty in assessing patient.

Indications for admission

- Confusion or reduced GCS.
- Abnormalities on imaging.
- Neurological signs or headache or vomiting.
- Difficulty in assessing patient.
- Coexisting medical problem.
- Inadequate social conditions or lack of responsible adult to observe patient.

Indications for neurosurgical referral

- Skull fracture + confusion/decreasing GCS.
- Focal neurological signs or fits.
- Persistence of neurological signs or confusion for >12 hours.
- Persisting coma (GCS ≤8) after resuscitation.
- Definite or suspected penetrating injury.
- Depressed skull fracture or CSF leak.
- Deterioration.

Severe head injury

- Patient will arrive unconscious in accident and emergency department. Head injury may be part of a multiple trauma.
- ABC (see Chapter 37). Intubate and ventilate unconscious patients to protect airway and prevent secondary brain injury from hypoxia.
- Resuscitate patient and look for other injuries, especially if the patient is in shock. Head injury may be accompanied by cervical spine injury and the neck must be protected by a cervical collar in these patients.
- Treat life-threatening problems (e.g. ruptured spleen) and stabilize patient before transfer to neurosurgical unit. Ensure adequate medical supervision (anaesthetist + nurse) during transfer.

Complications

Skull fractures

Indicate severity of injury. No specific treatment required unless compound, depressed or associated with chronic CSF loss (e.g. anterior cranial fossa basal skull fracture).

Intracranial haemorrhage

- Extradural haemorrhage: tear in middle meningeal artery. Haematoma between skull and dura. Often a 'lucid interval' before signs of raised ICP ensue (falling pulse, rising BP, ipsilateral pupillary dilatation, contralateral paresis or paralysis). Treatment is by evacuation of haematoma via burr holes.
- Acute subdural haemorrhage: tearing of veins between arachnoid and dura mater. Usually seen in elderly. Progressive neurological deterioration. Treatment is by evacuation but even then recovery may be incomplete.
- Chronic subdural haematoma: tear in vein leads to subdural haematoma which enlarges slowly by absorption of CSF. Often the precipitating injury is trivial. Drowsiness and confusion, headache, hemiplegia. Treatment is by evacuation of the clot.
- Intracerebral haemorrhage: haemorrhage into brain substance causes irreversible damage. Efforts are made to avoid secondary injury by ensuring adequate oxygenation and nutrition.

Raised intracranial pressure

Cerebral oedema is an increase in brain volume caused by an absolute increase in cerebral water content and results in raised ICP. Frequently, raised ICP complicates closed head injury. Management may involve some of the following: ICP monitoring, head elevation, maintenance of cerebral perfusion, CSF drainage by ventriculostomy, hyperventilation, hypothermia, diuretics (mannitol), barbiturates and decompressive craniectomy.

Prognosis

Prognosis is related to level of consciousness on arrival in hospital.

GCS on admission	Mortality
15	1%
8–12	5%
<8	40%

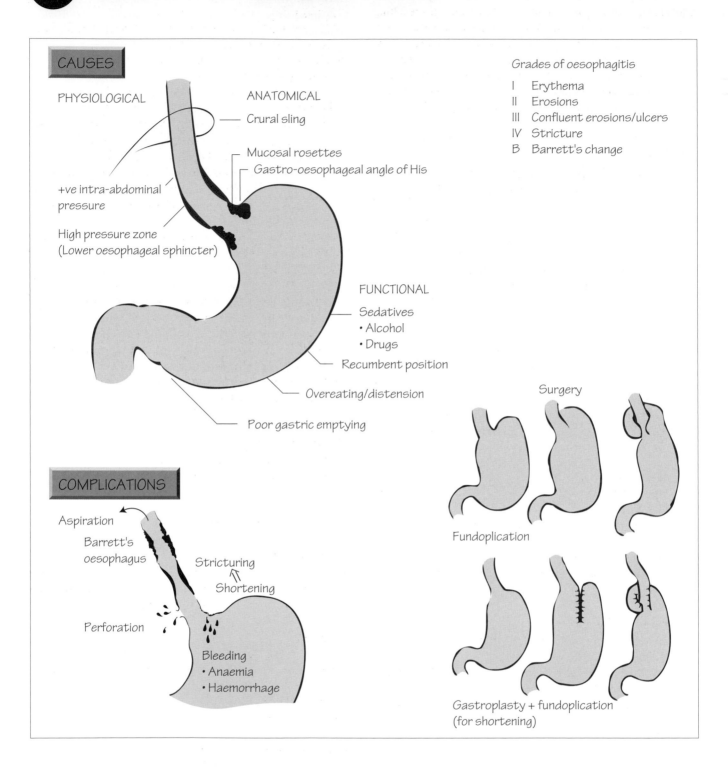

CAUSES

PHYSIOLOGICAL

ANATOMICAL

Crural sling

Mucosal rosettes

Gastro-oesophageal angle of His

+ve intra-abdominal pressure

High pressure zone (Lower oesophageal sphincter)

FUNCTIONAL

Sedatives
• Alcohol
• Drugs

Recumbent position

Overeating/distension

Poor gastric emptying

Grades of oesophagitis

I   Erythema
II Erosions
III Confluent erosions/ulcers
IV Stricture
B   Barrett's change

Surgery

Fundoplication

Gastroplasty + fundoplication
(for shortening)

COMPLICATIONS

Aspiration

Barrett's oesophagus

Stricturing

Shortening

Perforation

Bleeding
• Anaemia
• Haemorrhage

Definitions

Gastro-oesophageal reflux is a condition caused by the retrograde passage of gastric contents into the oesophagus resulting in inflammation (*oesophagitis*), which manifests as dyspepsia. A *hiatus hernia* is an abnormal protrusion of the proximal stomach through the oesophageal opening in the diaphragm resulting in a more proximal positioning of the oesophagogastric junction and predisposition to GORD. *Sliding* (common) and *rolling* or *para-oesophageal* (rare) hiatus hernias are recognized.

Key points

- The majority of GORD is benign and uncomplicated.
- Barrett's oesophagus is an increasingly recognized association predisposing to adenocarcinoma of the oesophagus.
- Patients over the age of 45 years or with suspicious symptoms should have malignancy excluded as a cause when first presenting with GORD symptoms.
- Surgery for GORD should be reserved for complications or patients resistant to medical therapy.

Common causes

- Failure of normal mechanisms of gastro-oesophageal continence (LOS pressure, length of intra-abdominal LOS, angle of His, sling fibres around the cardia, the crural fibres of the diaphragm, the mucosal rosette).
- LOS pressure reduced by smoking, alcohol and coffee and some drugs (calcium-channel blockers, nitrates, beta-blockers, progesterone).

Clinical features

- Retrosternal burning pain, radiating to epigastrium, jaw and arms. (Oesophageal pain is often confused with cardiac pain.)
- Regurgitation of acid contents into the mouth (waterbrash).
- Back pain (a penetrating ulcer in Barrett's oesophagus).
- Dysphagia from a benign stricture.
- Coughing or wheezing, hoarseness (due to aspiration of gastric contents).

Investigations

- Barium swallow and meal: sliding hiatus hernia, oesophageal ulcer, stricture.
- Oesophagoscopy: assess oesophagitis, biopsy for histology, dilate stricture if present.
- Ambulatory 24-hour pH monitoring: assess the degree of reflux.
- Oesophageal manometry.

Essential management

General

- Lose weight, avoid smoking, coffee, alcohol, chocolate, tomatoes and citrus juices.
- Avoid tight garments and stooping. Avoid large meals. Elevate head of bed.

Medical

- Exclude carcinoma by OGD in patients over 45 years and with symptoms suspicious of malignancy.
- Control acid secretion (H_2 receptor antagonists (e.g. ranitidine) or PPIs (e.g. omeprazole)). Antacids may be effective in controlling symptoms in mild disease.
- Minimize effects of reflux (give alginates to protect oesophagus).
- Prokinetic agents (e.g. metoclopramide, cisapride) improve LOS tone and promote gastric emptying.

Surgical

- Antireflux surgery (e.g. Nissen fundoplication) which may be performed by laparotomy or laparoscopy. Indicated in approximately 20% of patients with GORD with:
  - complications of reflux (stricture, Barrret's oesophagus)
  - failed medical control of symptoms
  - ?long-term dependence on medical treatment
  - ?'large volume' reflux

Complications

- Benign stricture of the oesophagus.
- Barrett's oesophagus (see below).
- Bleeding.

Barrett's oesophagus

Definition and aetiology

3 cm of columnar epithelium lining the lower anatomical oesophagus. May be related to eradication of *Helicobacter pylori* and increasing incidence of GORD.

Diagnosis

Can only be confidently made by biopsy but appearances of 'reddish' mucosa in the lower oesophagus are typical on OGD.

Complications

Risk of adenocarcinoma:
- 2%—no dysplasia present.
- 20%—low-grade dysplasia present.
- 50%—high-grade dysplasia present.

Treatment

- Follow-up OGD (close surveillance if low-grade dysplasia) and PPIs.
- Possibly laparoscopic fundoplication.
- Oesophagectomy if high-grade dysplasia due to risk of carcinoma.

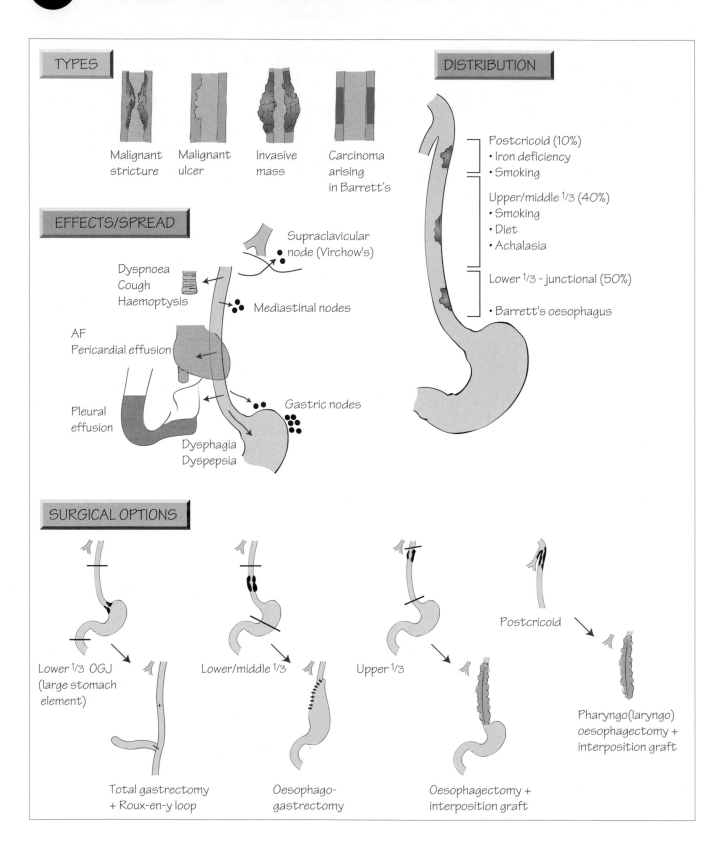

TYPES

Malignant stricture

Malignant ulcer

Invasive mass

Carcinoma arising in Barrett's

DISTRIBUTION

Postcricoid (10%)
• Iron deficiency
• Smoking

Upper/middle 1/3 (40%)
• Smoking
• Diet
• Achalasia

Lower 1/3 - junctional (50%)

• Barrett's oesophagus

EFFECTS/SPREAD

Supraclavicular node (Virchow's)

Dyspnoea
Cough
Haemoptysis

Mediastinal nodes

AF
Pericardial effusion

Pleural effusion

Gastric nodes

Dysphagia
Dyspepsia

SURGICAL OPTIONS

Lower 1/3 OGJ (large stomach element)

Total gastrectomy + Roux-en-y loop

Lower/middle 1/3

Oesophago-gastrectomy

Upper 1/3

Oesophagectomy + interposition graft

Postcricoid

Pharyngo(laryngo) oesophagectomy + interposition graft

Definition

Malignant lesion of the epithelial lining of the oesophagus.

> ### Key points
>
> - All new symptoms of dysphagia should raise the possibility of oesophageal carcinoma.
> - Adenocarcinoma of the oesophagus is increasingly common.
> - Only a minority of tumours are successfully cured by surgery.

Epidemiology

- Male : female 3 : 1, peak incidence 50–70 years. High incidence in areas of China, Russia, Scandinavia and among the Bantu in South Africa.
- Adenocarcinoma has the fastest increasing incidence of any carcinoma in the UK.

Aetiology

Predisposing factors:
- Chronic oesophagitis and Barrett's oesophagus—possibly related to biliary reflux.
- Alcohol consumption and cigarette smoking.
- Stricture from corrosive (lye) oesophagitis.
- Achalasia.
- Plummer–Vinson syndrome (oesophageal web, mucosal lesions of mouth and pharynx, iron deficiency anaemia).
- Nitrosamines.

Pathology

- Histological type: 20% squamous carcinoma (upper two-thirds of oesophagus); 80% adenocarcinoma (middle third, lower third and junctional).
- Spread: lymphatics, direct extension, vascular invasion.

Clinical features

- Dysphagia progressing from solids to liquids.
- Weight loss and weakness.
- Aspiration pneumonia.

Investigations

- Oesophagoscopy and biopsy (minimum of eight biopsies): malignant stricture.
- Barium swallow (if high lesion suspected or OGD contraindicated): narrowed lumen with 'shouldering'.
- Bronchoscopy: assess if bronchial invasion suspected with upper third lesions.
- EUS: useful in staging disease (depth of penetration [T staging] and perioesophageal nodes [N staging]).
- Contrast enhanced abdominal and chest CT scanning/MRI: assess degree of spread if surgery is being contemplated—especially metastases (M staging).

- PET scanning: increasingly used.
- Laparoscopy to assess liver and peritoneal involvement prior to proceeding to surgery.

> ### Essential management
>
> #### Palliation
>
> - Partially covered self-expanding metal stents are the intubation of choice for obstructive symptoms—especially useful when tracheo-oesophageal fistula present ± laser therapy.
> - Radiotherapy—external beam DXT or endoluminal brachytherapy.
> - Laser resection (Nd:YAG laser) of the tumour to create lumen.
> - Photodynamic therapy: photosensitizing agents are taken up by dysplastic malignant tissue which is damaged when photons (light) is applied.
>
> #### Curative treatment
>
> - Surgical resection is potentially curative only if lymph nodes are not involved and clear tumours margins can be achieved.
> - Neoadjuvant (pre-operative) or adjuvant (postoperative) treatment (chemotherapy or chemoradiotherapy) is not recommended now outside clinical trials.
> - Chemoradiotherapy and radiotherapy are occasionally used with curative intent in patients deemed not suitable for surgery.
> - Reconstruction is by jejunal or gastric 'pull-up' or rarely colon interposition.

Prognosis

Following resection, 5-year survival rates are about 15%, but overall 5-year survival (palliation and resection) is only about 4%.

> ### 2 Week wait referral criteria for suspected upper GI cancer
>
> - New-onset dysphagia (any age).
> - Dyspepsia + 'alarm symptoms': weight loss/anaemia/vomiting.
> - Dyspepsia + FHx/Barrett's oesophagus/previous peptic ulcer surgery/atrophic gastritis/pernicious anaemia.
> - New dyspepsia >55 years.
> - Jaundice.
> - Upper abdominal mass.

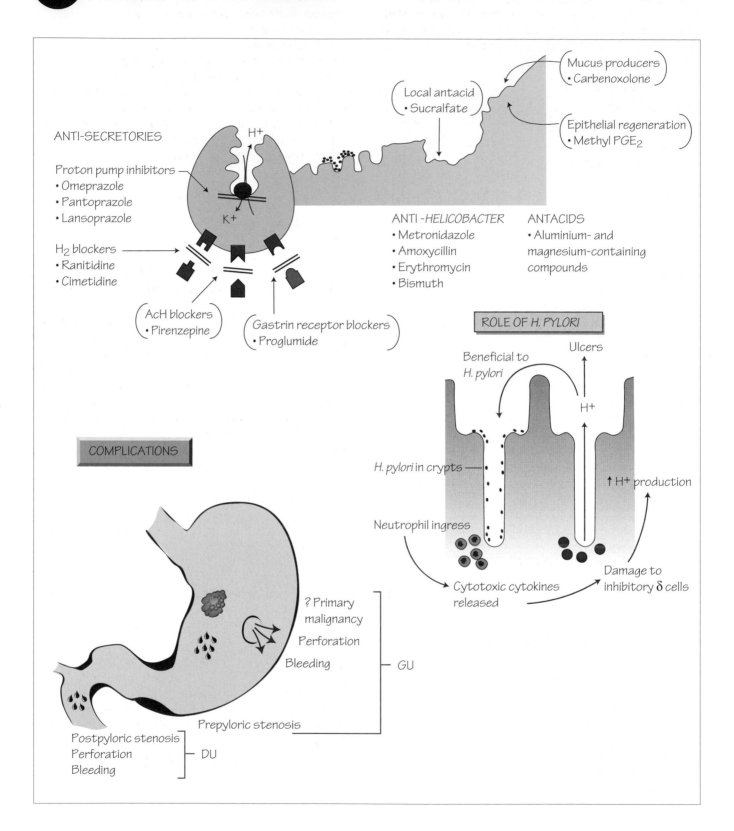

ANTI-SECRETORIES

Proton pump inhibitors
• Omeprazole
• Pantoprazole
• Lansoprazole

H$_2$ blockers
• Ranitidine
• Cimetidine

AcH blockers
• Pirenzepine

Gastrin receptor blockers
• Proglumide

Local antacid
• Sucralfate

Mucus producers
• Carbenoxolone

Epithelial regeneration
• Methyl PGE$_2$

ANTI-HELICOBACTER
• Metronidazole
• Amoxycillin
• Erythromycin
• Bismuth

ANTACIDS
• Aluminium- and magnesium-containing compounds

ROLE OF H. PYLORI

Beneficial to H. pylori

Ulcers

H$^+$

H. pylori in crypts

↑ H$^+$ production

Neutrophil ingress

Damage to inhibitory δ cells

Cytotoxic cytokines released

COMPLICATIONS

? Primary malignancy

Perforation

Bleeding

GU

Prepyloric stenosis

Postpyloric stenosis
Perforation
Bleeding

DU

Definition

A *peptic ulcer* is a break in the epithelial surface of the oesophagus, stomach or duodenum (rarely Meckel's diverticulum) caused by the action of gastric secretions (acid and pepsin) and, in the case of duodenal ulceration, infection with *Helicobacter pylori*.

Key points

- Not all dyspepsia is due to PUD.
- The majority of chronic duodenal ulcers are related to *H. pylori* infection and respond to eradication therapy.
- All patients over 45 years at presentation or with suspicious symptoms require endoscopy to exclude malignancy.
- Surgery is limited to complications of ulcer disease.

Common causes

- Imbalance between acid/pepsin secretion and mucosal defence.
- Acid hypersecretion occurs because of increased numbers of parietal cells (or rarely in response to gastrin hypersecretion in the Zollinger–Ellison syndrome or antral G cell hyperplasia).
- Defects in mucosal defence (e.g. mucus secretion).
- NSAIDs and the usual suspects: alcohol, cigarettes and 'stress'.
- Infection with *H. pylori*.

Clinical features

Duodenal ulcer and type II gastric ulcer (i.e. prepyloric and antral)

- Male : female 1 : 1, peak incidence 25–50 years.
- Epigastric pain during fasting (hunger pain), relieved by food/antacids, often nocturnal, typically exhibits periodicity (i.e. recurs at regular intervals).
- Boring back pain if ulcer is penetrating posteriorly.
- Haematemesis from ulcer penetrating gastroduodenal artery posteriorly.
- Peritonitis if perforation occurs with anterior DU.
- Vomiting if gastric outlet obstruction (pyloric stenosis) occurs (note succussion splash and watch for hypokalaemic, hypochloraemic alkalosis).

Type I gastric ulcer (i.e. body of stomach)

- Male : female 3 : 1, peak incidence 50+ years.
- Epigastric pain induced by eating.
- Weight loss.
- Nausea and vomiting.
- Anaemia from chronic blood loss.

Investigations

- FBC: to check for anaemia.
- U+E: rarely indicates Zollinger–Ellison syndrome.
- Faecal occult blood.
- OGD: necessary to exclude malignant gastric ulcer in:
  patients over 45 years at first presentation
  concomitant anaemia
  short history of symptoms
  other 'alarm' symptoms suggestive of malignancy
- Useful to obtain biopsy for CLO and rapid urease test.
- Barium meal: best for patients unable to tolerate OGD or evaluation of the duodenum in cases of pyloric stenosis.
- Carbon 13-urease breath test/*H. pylori* serology: non-invasive method of assessing the presence of *H. pylori* infection. Used to direct therapy or confirm eradication.

Essential management

Medical

Triple therapy:
- *H. pylori* should be eradicated to facilitate healing and reduce risk of recurrence (Rx 250 mg clarithromycin + 400 mg metronidazole *or* 1 g amoxicillin 500 mg clarithromycin b.i.d. for 7 days) *and*
- Full dose PPIs (20 mg omeprazole or 30 mg lansoprazole b.i.d.) for suppression of acid secretion for 7 days.
- NSAID-induced ulcers: PPIs—4 weeks for DU, 8 weeks for GU.
- Re-endoscope patients with GU after 6 weeks because of risk of malignancy.
- Patient with complication (bleeding perforation) should undergo *H. pylori* eradication.

Other therapy:
- Avoid smoking and foods that cause pain.
- Avoid NSAIDs.
- Antacids for symptomatic relief.
- H_2 blockers (ranitidine, cimetidine).
- Colloidal bismuth may be used with metronidazole and tetracycline for *H. pylori* eradication.

Surgical

- Only indicated for failure of medical treatment and complications.
- Elective for DU: highly selective vagotomy; rarely performed now.
- Elective for GU: Billroth I gastrectomy.
- Perforated DU/GU: simple closure of perforation and biopsy (may be laparoscopic).
- Haemorrhage: endoscopic control by sclerotherapy/injection/haemoclips/heater probe, surgical—undersewing bleeding vessel.
- Pyloric stenosis: gastroenterostomy ± truncal vagotomy.

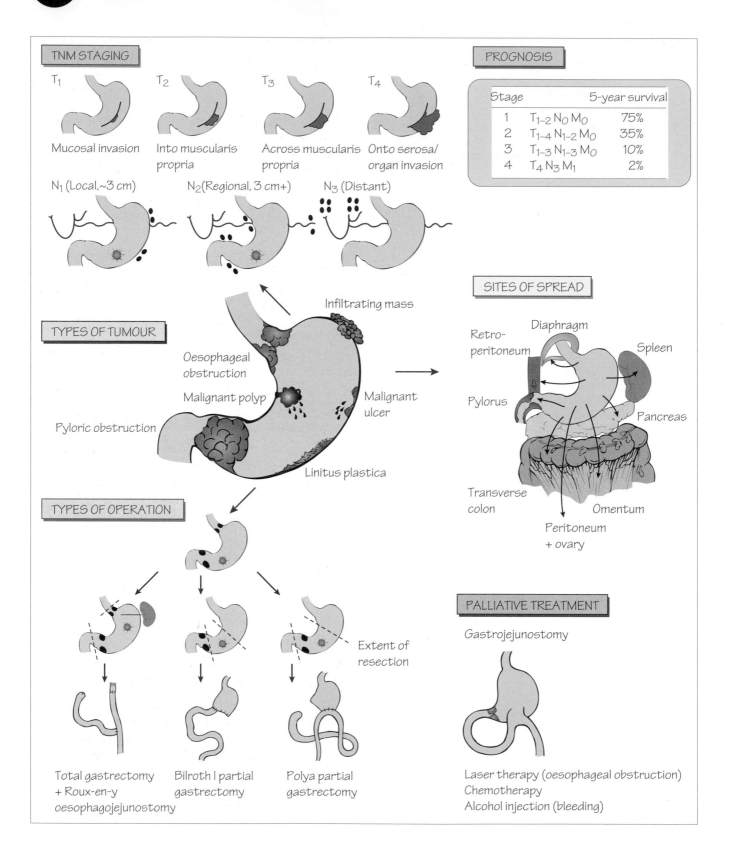

TNM STAGING

T_1 — Mucosal invasion

T_2 — Into muscularis propria

T_3 — Across muscularis propria

T_4 — Onto serosa/organ invasion

N_1 (Local, ~3 cm)

N_2 (Regional, 3 cm+)

N_3 (Distant)

PROGNOSIS

Stage		5-year survival
1	$T_{1-2} N_0 M_0$	75%
2	$T_{1-4} N_{1-2} M_0$	35%
3	$T_{1-3} N_{1-3} M_0$	10%
4	$T_4 N_3 M_1$	2%

TYPES OF TUMOUR

Infiltrating mass

Oesophageal obstruction

Malignant polyp

Pyloric obstruction

Malignant ulcer

Linitus plastica

SITES OF SPREAD

Retro-peritoneum

Diaphragm

Spleen

Pylorus

Pancreas

Transverse colon

Omentum

Peritoneum + ovary

TYPES OF OPERATION

Extent of resection

Total gastrectomy + Roux-en-y oesophagojejunostomy

Bilroth I partial gastrectomy

Polya partial gastrectomy

PALLIATIVE TREATMENT

Gastrojejunostomy

Laser therapy (oesophageal obstruction)
Chemotherapy
Alcohol injection (bleeding)

Definition

Malignant lesion of the stomach epithelium.

Key points

- Second most common cause of cancer-related death worldwide.
- The majority of tumours are unresectable at presentation.
- Tumours considered candidates for resection should be staged with CT and laparoscopy to reduce the risk of an 'open and shut' laparotomy.
- Most tumours are poorly responsive to chemotherapy.

Epidemiology

Male : female 2 : 1, peak incidence 50+ years. Associated with poor socioeconomic status. Dramatic difference in incidence according to geography/genetics (population). Incidence has decreased in Western world over last 50 years. Still common in Japan, Chile and Scandinavia.

Aetiology

Predisposing factors:
- *H. pylori*: two- to threefold increase of gastric cancer in infected individuals (*H. pylori* infection of the stomach reduces risk of oesophageal *adeno*carcinoma).
- Diet (smoked fish, pickled vegetables, benzpyrene, nitrosamines), smoking, alcohol.
- Atrophic gastritis, pernicious anaemia, previous partial gastrectomy.
- Familial hypogammaglobulinaemia.
- Positive family history (possibly related to E-cadherin gene mutation).
- Blood group A.

Pathology

- Histology: adenocarcinoma.
- Advanced gastric cancer (penetrated muscularis propria) may be polypoid, ulcerating or infiltrating (i.e. linitus plastica).
- Early gastric cancer (confined to mucosa or submucosa).
- Spread: lymphatic (e.g. Troisier's sign in Virchow's node); haematogenous to liver, lung, brain; transcoelomic to ovary (Krukenberg tumour).

Clinical features

- Dyspepsia (epigastric discomfort, postprandial fullness, loss of appetite).
- Anaemia.
- Dysphagia.
- Vomiting.
- Anorexia and weight loss.
- The presence of physical signs usually indicates advanced (incurable) disease.

Investigations

- FBC.
- U+E.
- LFTs.
- OGD (see the lesion and obtain biopsy to distinguish from benign gastric ulcer).
- Barium meal (space-occupying lesion/ulcer with rolled edge). Best for patients unable to tolerate OGD. Less sensitive than OGD for detecting early malignancy.
- CT scan (helical)/MRI: stages disease locally and systemically.
- PET scanning: no advantage over standard imaging in locating occult metastatic disease.
- Endoscopic ultrasound: more accurate than CT for T and N staging.
- Laparoscopy: used to exclude undiagnosed peritoneal or liver secondaries prior to consideration of resection.

Essential management

- Palliation (metastatic disease or gross distal nodal disease at presentation):
  intubation with self-expanding metal stents: obstructing lesions at the cardia or the gastric outlet
  palliative gastrectomy: only for local symptoms, e.g. bleeding
  laparoscopic gastroenterostomy: malignant gastric outlet obstruction
- Palliative chemotherapy: consider cisplatin and 5-FU to improve quality of life.
- Curative treatment (resectable primary and local nodes).
- Surgical principles are excision with clear margins and locoregional lymph node clearance (e.g. D2 gastrectomy).
- Other treatment: combination chemotherapy with etoposide, adriamycin and cisplatin may induce regression.

Prognosis

Following 'curative' resection, 5-year survival rates are approximately 20%, but overall 5-year survival (palliation and resection) is only about 5%.

2 Week wait referral criteria for suspected upper GI cancer

- New-onset dysphagia (any age).
- Dyspepsia + weight loss/anaemia/vomiting.
- Dyspepsia + FHx/Barrett's oesophagus/previous peptic ulcer surgery/atrophic gastritis/pernicious anaemia.
- New dyspepsia >55 years.
- Jaundice.
- Upper abdominal mass.

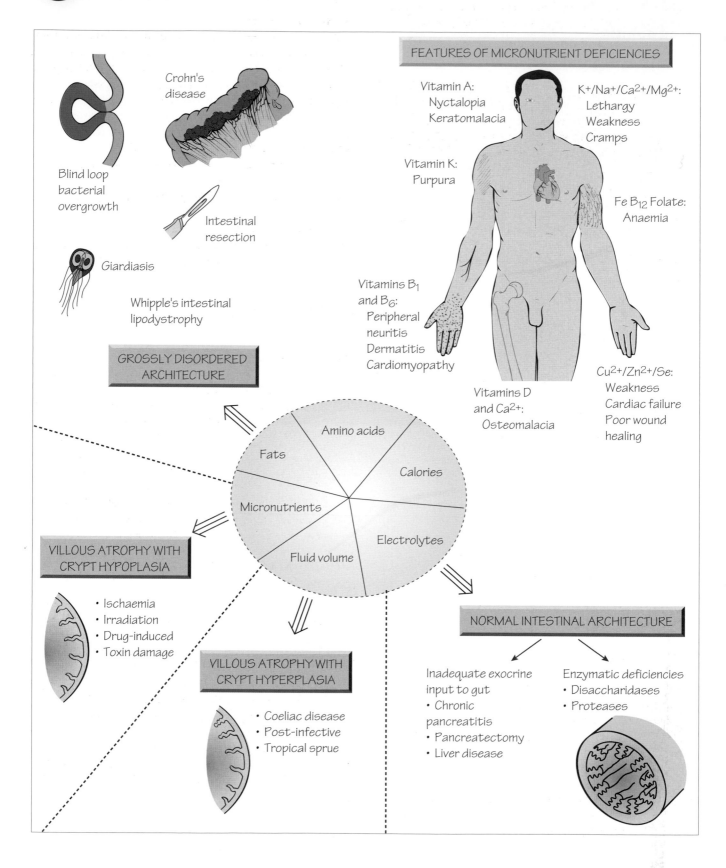

Crohn's disease

Blind loop bacterial overgrowth

Intestinal resection

Giardiasis

Whipple's intestinal lipodystrophy

GROSSLY DISORDERED ARCHITECTURE

FEATURES OF MICRONUTRIENT DEFICIENCIES

Vitamin A:
Nyctalopia
Keratomalacia

$K^+/Na^+/Ca^{2+}/Mg^{2+}$:
Lethargy
Weakness
Cramps

Vitamin K:
Purpura

Fe B_{12} Folate:
Anaemia

Vitamins B_1 and B_6:
Peripheral neuritis
Dermatitis
Cardiomyopathy

Vitamins D and Ca^{2+}:
Osteomalacia

$Cu^{2+}/Zn^{2+}/Se$:
Weakness
Cardiac failure
Poor wound healing

Amino acids

Fats

Calories

Micronutrients

Electrolytes

Fluid volume

VILLOUS ATROPHY WITH CRYPT HYPOPLASIA

- Ischaemia
- Irradiation
- Drug-induced
- Toxin damage

VILLOUS ATROPHY WITH CRYPT HYPERPLASIA

- Coeliac disease
- Post-infective
- Tropical sprue

NORMAL INTESTINAL ARCHITECTURE

Inadequate exocrine input to gut
- Chronic pancreatitis
- Pancreatectomy
- Liver disease

Enzymatic deficiencies
- Disaccharidases
- Proteases

Definition

Malabsorption is the failure of the body to acquire and conserve adequate amounts of one or more essential dietary elements. Encompasses a series of defects occurring during the digestion and absorption of nutrients from the GI tract. The cause may be localized or generalized.

Key points

- Malabsorption usually affects several nutrient groups.
- Coeliac disease is a common cause and may present with obscure, vague abdominal symptoms.
- Always consider micronutrients and trace elements in malabsorption.

Clinical features

- Diarrhoea (often watery from increased osmotic load).
- Steatorrhoea (from fat malabsorption).
- Weight loss and fatigue.
- Flatulence and abdominal distension (bacterial action on undigested food products).
- Oedema (hypoalbuminaemia).
- Anaemia (Fe^{2+}, vitamin B_{12}), bleeding disorders (vitamin K, vitamin C), bone pain, pathological fracture (vitamin D, Ca^{2+}).
- Neurological (Ca^{2+}, Mg^{2+}, folic acid, vitamin A, vitamin B_{12}).

Differential diagnosis

Coeliac disease

- Classically presents as sensitivity to gluten-containing foods with diarrhoea, steatorrhoea and weight loss in early adulthood.
- Mild forms may present later in life with non-specific symptoms of malaise, anaemia (including iron deficiency picture), abdominal cramps and weight loss.

Crohn's disease

- Most common presenting symptoms are colicky abdominal pains with diarrhoea and weight loss.
- Malabsorption is an uncommon presenting symptom but often accompanies stenosing or inflammatory complications of widespread ileal disease.

Intestinal resection

- Global malabsorption may develop after small bowel resections leaving <50 cm of functional ileum. Water and electrolyte balance is most disordered but fat, vitamin and other nutrient absorption is also affected with lengths progressively <50 cm.
- Specific malabsorption may result from relatively small resection (e.g. fat and vitamin B_{12} malabsorption after terminal ileal resection, vitamin B_{12} and iron malabsorption after gastrectomy).

Whipple's disease (intestinal lipodystrophy)

- Fat malabsorption caused by intestinal infection blocking the lacteals with macrophages and bacteria.

- Presents with steatorrhoea associated with arthralgia and malaise.

Bacterial overgrowth

- Malabsorption caused by bacterial metabolism of nutrients and production of breakdown products such as CO_2 and H_2.
- Usually a result of exclusion of a loop of ileum (e.g. in Crohn's disease, postsurgery, intestinal fistulation) with consequent bacterial overgrowth, although can occur in chronically damaged or dilated bowel.

Radiation enteropathy

- Slow onset, progressive global malabsorption. Usually only if large areas of ileum affected.
- May occur many years after original radiotherapy exposure.

Chronic ischaemic enteropathy

Rare cause of malabsorption. Usually accompanied by chronic intestinal ischaemia causing 'mesenteric angina/claudication' upon eating.

Parasitic infection

Common in tropics but rare in the UK.

Investigations

- FBC, U+E, LFTs: general nutritional status.
- Trace elements (Zn, Se, Mg, Mn, Cu).
- 72-hour faecal fat collection (detects fat malabsorption).
- D-xylose test (integrity of intestinal mucosa).
- Hydrogen (lactase deficiency) and bile salt (bile salt metabolism) breath tests.
- Schilling test (vitamin B_{12} deficiency)—intrinsic factor, pancreatic insufficiency, ileal resection/disease.
- Anti α-gliadin antibodies (serum assay for coeliac disease).
- Small bowel meal or enema: best for Crohn's disease, radiation or ischaemic enteropathy and blind loop formation.
- Upper GI endoscopy and small bowel biopsy

Essential management

- Major deficiencies should be corrected by supplementation (oral or parenteral).
- Infectious causes should be excluded or (consider probiotics) treated promptly.
- Coeliac disease: gluten-free diet.
- Crohn's disease: usually requires resection of affected segment. Course of systemic steroids or immunosuppressive agents may help.
- Radiation or ischaemic malabsorption rarely responds to any medical therapy—often requires parenteral nutrition.

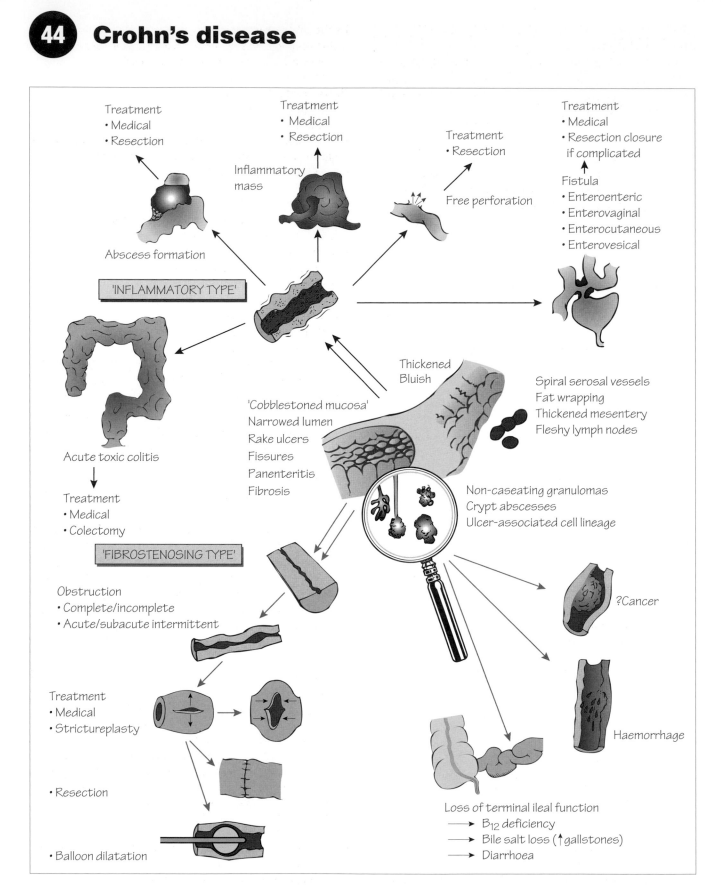

Treatment
• Medical
• Resection

Treatment
• Medical
• Resection

Treatment
• Resection

Treatment
• Medical
• Resection closure
  if complicated

Fistula
• Enteroenteric
• Enterovaginal
• Enterocutaneous
• Enterovesical

Inflammatory
mass

Free perforation

Abscess formation

'INFLAMMATORY TYPE'

Thickened
Bluish

Spiral serosal vessels
Fat wrapping
Thickened mesentery
Fleshy lymph nodes

'Cobblestoned mucosa'
Narrowed lumen
Rake ulcers
Fissures
Panenteritis
Fibrosis

Acute toxic colitis

Treatment
• Medical
• Colectomy

'FIBROSTENOSING TYPE'

Non-caseating granulomas
Crypt abscesses
Ulcer-associated cell lineage

Obstruction
• Complete/incomplete
• Acute/subacute intermittent

?Cancer

Treatment
• Medical
• Strictureplasty

• Resection

Haemorrhage

• Balloon dilatation

Loss of terminal ileal function
⟶ B$_{12}$ deficiency
⟶ Bile salt loss (↑gallstones)
⟶ Diarrhoea

Definition

Crohn's disease is a chronic transmural inflammatory disorder of unknown cause affecting the predominantly the alimentary tract (any part from mouth to anus). Crohn's disease and ulcerative colitis together are referred to as *idiopathic inflammatory bowel disease*.

Epidemiology

Male : female 1 : 1.6. Young adults. High incidence among Europeans and Jewish people. Family tendency to the disease (multiple genetic associations identified).

Aetiology

- Unknown.
- Impaired cell-mediated immunity.
- Genetic link probable but candidate genes unknown (a gene called *NOD2* possibly involved).
- No proven link to mycobacterial infection or measles virus hypersensitivity.
- Smoking associated with recurrence (particularly in young women).

Pathology
Macroscopic

- May affect any part of the alimentary tract.
- Skip lesions in bowel (affected bowel wall and mesentery are thickened and oedematous, frequent fistulae).
- Affected bowel characteristically 'fat wrapped' by mesenteric fat.
- Perianal disease characterized by perianal induration (blue skin discoloration) and sepsis with fissure, sinus and fistula formation.

Histology

- Transmural inflammation in the form of lymphoid aggregates.
- Non-caseating epithelioid cell granulomas with Langhans giant cells. Regional nodes may also be involved.

Clinical features
Acute presentations (uncommon)

- RIF peritonitis (like appendicitis picture).
- Generalized peritonitis (due to free perforation).
- Acute colitis: uncommon as primary presentation.

Subacute presentations (common)

- RIF inflammatory mass (usually associated with fistulae or abscess formation).
- Widespread ileal inflammation: general ill health, malnutrition, anaemia, abdominal pain.
- Colitis: abdominal pain and bloody diarrhoea.

Chronic presentations

- Strictures: intermittent colicky abdominal pains associated with eating—'food fear'.
- Malabsorption (due to widespread disease often with previous resections).
- Growth retardation in children (due to chronic malnutrition and chronic inflammatory response suppressing growth).

Perianal disease

- Up to one-third of patients may have perianal disease.
- Fissure *in ano*, fistula *in ano*, perianal sepsis.

Extraintestinal features

- Eye: episcleritis, uveitis.
- Acute phase proteins, e.g. CRP.
- Joints: arthritis (sacroiliac joint arthritis, ankylosing spondylitis).
- Skin: erythema nodosum, pyoderma gangrenosum.
- Liver: sclerosing cholangitis, cirrhosis.

Investigations

- FBC: macrocytic anaemia, WBC raised, ESR raised.
- Acute phase proteins, e.g. CRP
- Small bowel enema: narrowed terminal ileum, 'string sign' of Kantor, stricture formation, fistulae.
- Abdominal ultrasound: RIF mass, abscess formation.
- CT scan: RIF mass, abscess formation.
- Colonoscopy for Crohn's colitis.
- Indium-labelled white-cell scan: areas of inflammation.
- Video capsule endoscopy.

Prognosis

- Crohn's disease is a chronic problem, and recurrent episodes of active disease are common.
- 75% of patients will require surgery at some time.
- 60% of patients will require more than one operation.
- Life expectancy of Crohn's disease patients is little different from the 'normal' population.

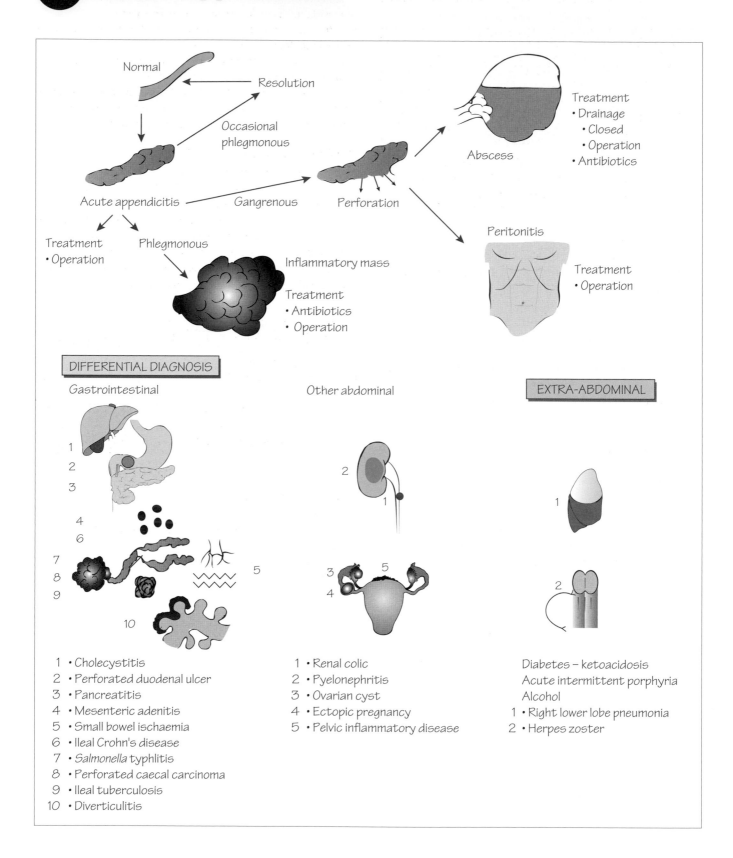

Normal

Resolution

Occasional
phlegmonous

Acute appendicitis

Gangrenous

Perforation

Abscess

Treatment
• Drainage
  • Closed
  • Operation
• Antibiotics

Treatment
• Operation

Phlegmonous

Inflammatory mass

Treatment
• Antibiotics
• Operation

Peritonitis

Treatment
• Operation

DIFFERENTIAL DIAGNOSIS

Gastrointestinal

Other abdominal

EXTRA-ABDOMINAL

1 • Cholecystitis
2 • Perforated duodenal ulcer
3 • Pancreatitis
4 • Mesenteric adenitis
5 • Small bowel ischaemia
6 • Ileal Crohn's disease
7 • *Salmonella* typhlitis
8 • Perforated caecal carcinoma
9 • Ileal tuberculosis
10 • Diverticulitis

1 • Renal colic
2 • Pyelonephritis
3 • Ovarian cyst
4 • Ectopic pregnancy
5 • Pelvic inflammatory disease

Diabetes – ketoacidosis
Acute intermittent porphyria
Alcohol
1 • Right lower lobe pneumonia
2 • Herpes zoster

Definition

Acute appendicitis is an inflammation of the vermiform appendix.

Key points

- 7 out of 10 cases of RIF pain in children under 10 years are non-specific and self-limiting.
- The most common differential diagnosis in young women is ovarian pathology.
- RIF peritonism over 55 years should raise the suspicion of other causes.
- Cross-sectional imaging (CT) should be obtained whenever there is real concern about the differential diagnosis to prevent inappropriate surgical exploration.

Epidemiology

Most common surgical emergency in the Western world. Rare under 2 years, common in second and third decades, but can occur at any age.

Pathology

- 'Obstructive': infection superimposed on luminal obstruction from any cause.
- 'Phlegmonous': viral infection, lymphoid hyperplasia, ulceration, bacterial invasion without obvious cause.
- 'Necrotic': usually secondary to obstructive causes with secondary infarction.

Clinical features

- Periumbilical abdominal pain, nausea, vomiting.
- Localization of pain to RIF.
- Mild pyrexia.
- Patient is flushed, tachycardia, furred tongue, halitosis.
- Tender (usually with rebound) over McBurney's point.
- Right-sided pelvic tenderness on PR examination.
- Peritonitis if appendix perforated.
- Appendix mass if patient presents late.

Investigations

- Diagnosis is a clinical diagnosis, but WCC (almost always leucocytosis) and CRP (usually raised) are helpful.
- Ultrasound for appendix mass and if in doubt to rule out other pelvic pathology (e.g. ovarian cyst).
- Laparoscopy commonly used to exclude ovarian pathology prior to appendicectomy in young women.
- CT scan (helical) in elderly patients or where other causes are considered possible. Most accurate non-invasive test for diagnosing appendicitis but requires significant radiation exposure.

Differential diagnosis

- Mesenteric lymphadenitis in children.
- Pelvic disease in women (e.g. PID, UTIs, ectopic pregnancy, ruptured corpus luteum cyst).
- More rarely: Crohn's disease, cholecystitis, perforated duodenal ulcer, right basal pneumonia, torsion of the right testis, diabetes mellitus in younger and middle-aged patients.
- Occasionally: perforated caecal carcinoma, sigmoid diverticulitis, caecal diverticulitis in elderly patients.

Essential management

- Acute appendicitis: appendicectomy, open or laparoscopic.
- Appendix mass: IV fluids, antibiotics, close observation. Then:
  - if symptoms resolve, interval appendicectomy after a few months
  - if symptoms progress, urgent appendicectomy ± drainage.

Complications

- Wound infection.
- Intra-abdominal abscess (pelvic, RIF, subphrenic).
- Adhesions.
- Abdominal actinomycosis (rare).
- Portal pyaemia.

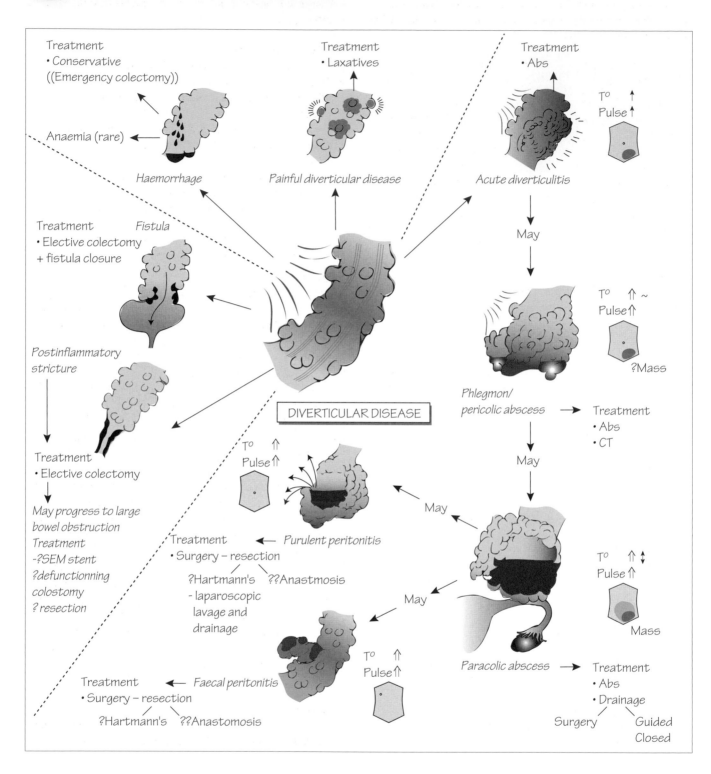

Treatment
• Conservative
((Emergency colectomy))

Anaemia (rare)

Haemorrhage

Treatment
• Laxatives

Painful diverticular disease

Treatment
• Abs

T⁰ ↑
Pulse ↑

Acute diverticulitis

May

Treatment   *Fistula*
• Elective colectomy
+ fistula closure

*Postinflammatory
stricture*

Treatment
• Elective colectomy

May progress to large
bowel obstruction
Treatment
-?SEM stent
?defunctionning
colostomy
? resection

T⁰ ↑↑ ~
Pulse ↑↑

?Mass

*Phlegmon/
pericolic abscess* → Treatment
• Abs
• CT

May

DIVERTICULAR DISEASE

T⁰ ↑
Pulse ↑↑

Treatment   ← *Purulent peritonitis*
• Surgery – resection
    ?Hartmann's ??Anastmosis
    - laparoscopic
    lavage and
    drainage

May

May

T⁰ ↑↑ ↕
Pulse ↑↑

Mass

Paracolic abscess → Treatment
• Abs
• Drainage
  Surgery   Guided
               Closed

Treatment   ← *Faecal peritonitis*
• Surgery – resection
    ?Hartmann's   ??Anastomosis

T⁰ ↑
Pulse ↑↑

Definition

Diverticular disease (or diverticulosis) is a condition in which many sac-like mucosal projections (diverticula) develop in the large bowel, especially the sigmoid colon. Acute inflammation of a diverticulum causes *diverticulitis*.

Key points

- Most diverticular disease is asymptomatic.
- The majority of acute attacks are resolved by non-surgical treatment.
- Emergency surgery for complications has a high morbidity and mortality and often involves an intestinal stoma.
- Elective surgery should be reserved for recurrent proven symptoms and complications (e.g. stricture).
- 'Diverticular' strictures should be biopsied in case of underlying colon carcinoma.

Epidemiology

Male : female 1 : 1.5, peak incidence 40s and 50s onwards. High incidence in the Western world where it is found in 50% of people over 60 years.

Aetiology

- Low fibre in the diet causes an increase in intraluminal colonic pressure, resulting in herniation of the mucosa through the muscle coats of the wall of the colon.
- Weak areas in wall of colon where nutrient arteries penetrate to submucosa and mucosa.

Pathology
Macroscopic

- Diverticula mostly found in (thickened) sigmoid colon.
- Emerge between the taenia coli and may contain faecoliths.

Histological

Projections are *acquired diverticula* as they contain only mucosa, submucosa and serosa and not all layers of intestinal wall.

Clinical features

- Mostly asymptomatic.
- Painful diverticulosis: LIF pain, constipation, diarrhoea.
- Acute diverticulitis: malaise, fever, LIF pain and tenderness ± palpable mass and abdominal distension.
- Perforation: peritonitis + features of diverticulitis.
- Large bowel obstruction: absolute constipation, distension, colicky abdominal pain and vomiting.

- Fistula: to bladder (cystitis/pneumaturia/recurrent UTIs); to vagina (faecal discharge PV); to small intestine (diarrhoea).
- Lower GI bleed: painless spontaneous—distinguish from angiodysplasia.

Investigations

- Diverticulosis: barium enema (colonoscopy).
- Diverticulitis: FBC, WCC, U+E, chest X-ray, CT scan.
- ? Diverticular mass/paracolic abscess: CT scan.
- ? Perforation: plain film of abdomen, CT scan.
- ? Obstruction: gastrograffin or dilute barium enema, colonoscopy to exclude underlying malignancy.
- ? Fistula:
  colovesical: MSU, cystoscopy, barium enema, CT
  colovaginal: colposcopy, flexible sigmoidoscopy, CT
- Haemorrhage: colonoscopy, selective angiography.

Essential management

Medical
Painful or asymptomatic
High-fibre diet (fruit, vegetables, wholemeal breads, bran). Increase fluid intake.

Acute diverticulitis
- Antibiotics and bowel rest.
- Radiologically guided drainage for localized abscess.

Surgical
- Usually for complications/recurrent, proven acute attacks or failed medical treatment.
- Elective surgery without peritonitis: resect diseased colon and rejoin the ends (primary anastomosis) may be laparoscopic.
- Emergency left colon surgery with *diffuse* peritonitis: resect diseased segment, oversew distal bowel (i.e. upper rectum) and bring out proximal bowel as end-colostomy (Hartmann's procedure).
- Emergency left colon surgery with *limited or no* peritonitis: laparoscopic peritoneal lavage and drainage or resect diseased segment and rejoin the ends (primary anastomosis) with defunctioning proximal stoma.
- Complicated left colon surgery (e.g. colovesical fistula): resection, primary anastomosis (may have defunctioning proximal stoma) may be laparoscopic.

Prognosis

Diverticular disease is a 'benign' condition, but there is significant mortality and morbidity from the complications.

Ulcerative colitis

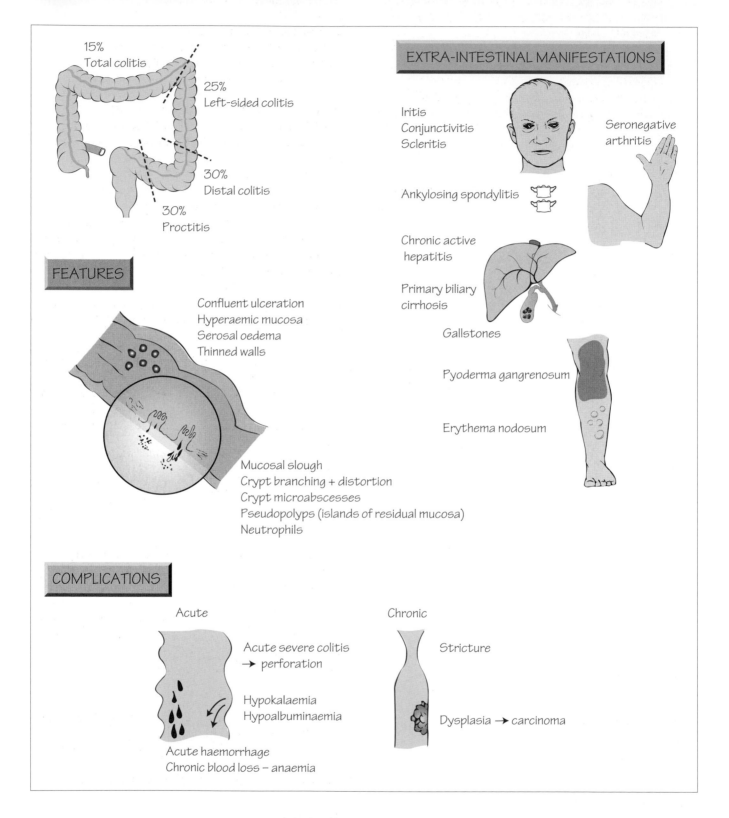

15%
Total colitis

25%
Left-sided colitis

30%
Distal colitis

30%
Proctitis

FEATURES

Confluent ulceration
Hyperaemic mucosa
Serosal oedema
Thinned walls

Mucosal slough
Crypt branching + distortion
Crypt microabscesses
Pseudopolyps (islands of residual mucosa)
Neutrophils

EXTRA-INTESTINAL MANIFESTATIONS

Iritis
Conjunctivitis
Scleritis

Seronegative
arthritis

Ankylosing spondylitis

Chronic active
 hepatitis

Primary biliary
cirrhosis

Gallstones

Pyoderma gangrenosum

Erythema nodosum

COMPLICATIONS

Acute

Acute severe colitis
→ perforation

Hypokalaemia
Hypoalbuminaemia

Acute haemorrhage
Chronic blood loss – anaemia

Chronic

Stricture

Dysplasia → carcinoma

Definition
A chronic inflammatory disorder of unknown cause of the colonic mucosa, usually beginning in the rectum and extending proximally to a variable extent. Ulcerative colitis and Crohn's disease together are referred to as *idiopathic inflammatory bowel disease*.

Epidemiology

Male : female 1 : 1.6, peak incidence 30–50 years. High incidence among relatives of patients (up to 40%) and among Europeans and people of Jewish descent.

Aetiology

- Genetic origin: increased prevalence (10%) in relatives, associated with HLA-B27 phenotype. Similar genes implicated in UC and Crohn's diease.
- May have autoimmune basis.
- Smoking protects against relapse.

Pathology

Disease confined to colon, rectum always involved, may be 'backwash' ileitis.

Macroscopic

In simple disease, only the mucosa is involved with superficial ulceration, exudation and pseudopolyposis. In severe disease, the full thickness of the colon wall may become involved in inflammation.

Histological

Mucin depletion, crypt abscess formation, acute neutrophilic infiltrate in severe disease, inflammatory pseudopolyps and highly vascular granulation tissue. Epithelial dysplasia with long-standing disease. (Sub)mucosal atrophy and fibrosis in chronic, 'burnt out' disease.

Clinical features

Proctitis

- Mucus, pus and blood PR.
- Urgency and frequency (diarrhoea less prominent).

Left-sided colitis → total colitis

Symptoms of proctitis + increasing features of systemic upset, abdominal pain, anorexia, weight loss and anaemia with more extensive disease.

Extraintestinal features

Percentage involved:
- Joints: arthritis (25%).
- Eye: uveitis (10%).
- Skin: erythema nodosum, pyoderma gangrenosum (10%).
- Liver: pericholangitis, fatty liver (3%), primary sclerosing cholangitis.
- Blood: thromboembolic disease (rare).

Severe/fulminant disease

- 6–20 bloody bowel motions per day/dehydration.
- Fever, anaemia, dehydration, electrolyte imbalance.
- Colonic dilatation/perforation—'toxic megacolon'/shock.

Investigations

- FBC: iron deficiency anaemia. WBC raised, ESR raised.
- Stool culture: including Crohn's disease toxin to exclude infective colitis before treatment.
- Plain abdominal radiograph: colonic dilatation or air under diaphragm indicating perforation in fulminant colitis.
- Barium enema: loss of haustrations, shortened 'lead pipe' colon.
- Sigmoidoscopy: inflamed friable mucosa, bleeds to touch.
- Colonoscopy: extent of disease at presentation, evaluation of response to treatment after exacerbations, screening of long-standing disease for dysplasia.
- Biopsy: typical histological features.

Prognosis

Ulcerative colitis is a chronic problem that requires constant surveillance unless surgery, which is drastic but curative, is performed.

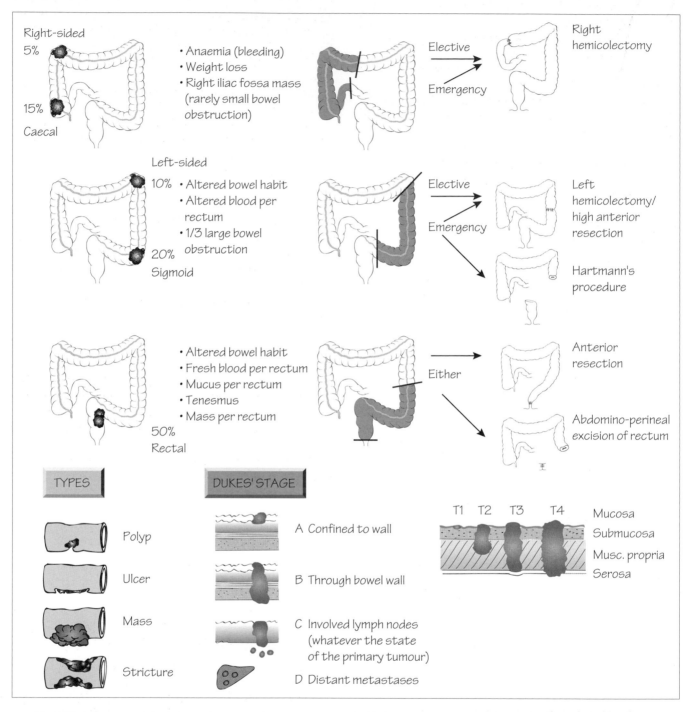

Right-sided
5%
15%
Caecal

- Anaemia (bleeding)
- Weight loss
- Right iliac fossa mass (rarely small bowel obstruction)

Elective
Emergency

Right hemicolectomy

Left-sided
10%
- Altered bowel habit
- Altered blood per rectum
- 1/3 large bowel obstruction
20%
Sigmoid

Elective
Emergency

Left hemicolectomy/ high anterior resection

Hartmann's procedure

- Altered bowel habit
- Fresh blood per rectum
- Mucus per rectum
- Tenesmus
- Mass per rectum
50%
Rectal

Either

Anterior resection

Abdomino-perineal excision of rectum

TYPES

Polyp
Ulcer
Mass
Stricture

DUKES' STAGE

A Confined to wall
B Through bowel wall
C Involved lymph nodes (whatever the state of the primary tumour)
D Distant metastases

T1 T2 T3 T4
Mucosa
Submucosa
Musc. propria
Serosa

Definition

Colorectal carcinoma (CRC) is the occurrence of malignant lesions in the mucosa of the colon ($^2/_3$) or rectum ($^1/_3$).

Key points

- Genetic factors have an important role in risk of CRC.
- Most colorectal cancers are left-sided and produce symptoms of bleeding or altered bowel habit.

- Prognosis depends mainly on stage at diagnosis.
- Surgery is the only curative treatment; radiotherapy and chemotherapy are both useful adjuncts.
- People should be treated by an MDT.
- National FOB-based screening programme likely to reduce mortality from CRC.
- 20% of patients with CRC present as emergencies.

Epidemiology

Male : female 1.3:1, peak incidence 50+ years increasing in the West.

Aetiology

Predisposing factors in decreasing importance:
- Prior CRC or adenomatous polyps.
- Hereditary syndromes (e.g. familial adenomatous polyposis, HNPCC, juvenile polyposis).
- Family history of CRC: 'population' lifetime risk of CRC 1 in 17, increasing risk with increasing number, low age and close relationship of affected relatives.
- Chronic active ulcerative colitis (see Chapter 47).
- Diet (low in indigestible fibre, high in animal fat).
- Increased faecal bile salts or folate deficiency.
- Regular NSAID usage reduces risk of CRC.

Pathology

Macroscopic
- Polypoid, ulcerating, annular, infiltrative.
- 75% of lesions are within rectum, sigmoid or left colon).
- 3% are synchronous (i.e. 2nd lesion found at the same time) and 3% are metachronous (i.e. 2nd lesion found later).

Histological
- Adenocarcinoma (10–15% are mucinous adenocarcinoma).
- Staging by Dukes' classification (A–D) and TNM.
- Spread: lymphatic (ly), haematogenous (v), peritoneal (peri).

Clinical features
- Anaemia—caecal cancers often present with anaemia.
- Colicky abdominal pain—tumours which are causing partial obstruction, e.g. transverse or descending colonic lesions.
- Alteration in bowel habit—either constipation or diarrhoea.
- Bleeding, passage of mucus PR, tenesmus (frequent or continuous desire to defaecate)—rectal tumour.

Investigations
- Digital rectal examination and faecal occult blood.
- FBC: anaemia.
- U+E: hypokalaemia, LFTs: liver metastases.
- Endoscopy: sigmoidoscopy (rigid to 30 cm/flexible to 60 cm) and colonoscopy (whole colon)—see the lesion, obtain biopsy.
- Double-contrast barium enema—'apple core lesion', polyp.
- CT colonography (via pneumocolon).
- CEA is often raised in advanced disease.

Essential management

Surgery (potentially curative)
Resection of the tumour with adequate margins to include regional lymph nodes is definitive treatment.

Procedures
- Resections may be open or laparoscopic, ± bowel preparation.
- Right hemicolectomy: lesions from caecum to hepatic flexure.

- Extended right hemicolectomy: lesions of the transverse colon.
- Left hemicolectomy (rare): lesions of the descending colon.
- Anterior resection excision for sigmoid colon and rectal tumours (total mesorectal excision for rectal tumours) ± proximal defunctioning stoma.
- Abdomino-perineal resection and colostomy for very low rectal lesions.
- Hartmann's procedure or resection with primary anastomosis for emergency surgery to left-sided colon tumours.
- Resection should be considered for liver or lung metastases if anatomically resectable with no evidence of other disseminated disease.
- Some rectal tumours are amenable to local excision (e.g. early T1, polyp cancer).

Surgery/interventions (palliative)
- Resection of the tumour (with anastomosis or stoma) for obstructing or symptomatic cancers despite metastases.
- Surgical bypass or defunctioning stoma for obstructing inoperable cancers.
- Transanal resection for symptomatic inoperable rectal cancer.
- Intraluminal stents for obstructing cancers.

Other treatment
- Radiotherapy; pre-operative 'neoadjuvant' to improve resectability and local control of potentially curable locally invasive rectal cancers, palliation of inoperable rectal cancer.
- Adjuvant chemotherapy (IV fluorouracil and folinic acid) is indicated for node or vascular invasion positive tumours—confers survival benefit.
- Palliative chemotherapy may be used to prolong survival in patients with unresectable metastases.

Prognosis
- 5-year survival depends on staging: A, 80%; B, 60%; C, 35%; D, 5%.
- 25% 5-year survival after successful resections of liver metastases.

2 Week wait referral criteria for suspected colorectal cancer
- Rectal bleeding + increased frequency or loose stools >6 weeks.
- Rectal bleeding without anal symptoms.
- Increased frequency or looser stools ?6 weeks.
- Rectal mass.
- Right-sided abdominal mass.
- Iron deficiency anaemia without obvious cause.

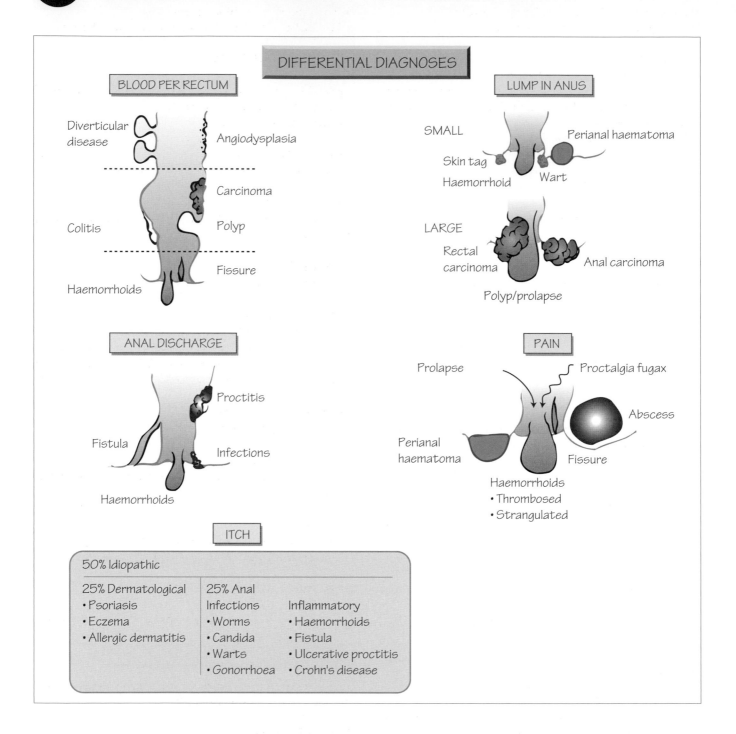

DIFFERENTIAL DIAGNOSES

BLOOD PER RECTUM

- Diverticular disease
- Angiodysplasia
- Carcinoma
- Colitis
- Polyp
- Fissure
- Haemorrhoids

LUMP IN ANUS

SMALL
- Skin tag
- Haemorrhoid
- Wart
- Perianal haematoma

LARGE
- Rectal carcinoma
- Anal carcinoma
- Polyp/prolapse

ANAL DISCHARGE

- Proctitis
- Fistula
- Infections
- Haemorrhoids

PAIN

- Prolapse
- Proctalgia fugax
- Abscess
- Perianal haematoma
- Fissure
- Haemorrhoids
  - Thrombosed
  - Strangulated

ITCH

50% Idiopathic

25% Dermatological	25% Anal	
• Psoriasis	Infections	Inflammatory
• Eczema	• Worms	• Haemorrhoids
• Allergic dermatitis	• Candida	• Fistula
	• Warts	• Ulcerative proctitis
	• Gonorrhoea	• Crohn's disease

Haemorrhoids ('piles')

Definition

A submucosal swelling in the anal canal consisting of a dilated venous plexus, a small artery and areolar tissue. Internal: only involves tissue of upper anal canal. External: involves tissue of lower anal canal.

Aetiology

- Increased venous pressure from straining (low-fibre diet) or altered haemodynamics (e.g. during pregnancy) causes chronic dilation of submucosal venous plexus.
- Found at the 3, 7 and 11 o'clock positions in the anal canal.

Clinical features

- First degree (1°): bleeding/itching only.
- Second degree (2°): prolapse during defaecation.
- Third degree (3°): constantly prolapsed.

Treatment

- Simple treatment—bulk laxatives and high-fibre diet.
- Bleeding internal piles—injection sclerotherapy, Barron's bands, cryosurgery, stapled haemorrhoidectomy (for circumferential and prolapsing).
- Prolapsing external—haemorrhoidectomy (complications: bleeding, anal stenosis).

Rectal prolapse

Definition

The protrusion from the anus to a variable degree of the rectal mucosa (partial) or rectal wall (full thickness).

Aetiology

Rectal intussusception, poor sphincter tone, chronic straining, pelvic floor injury.

Clinical features

Faecal incontinence, constipation, mucous discharge, bleeding, tenesmus, obvious prolapse. 10% of children with prolapse have cystic fibrosis.

Treatment

Stool manipulation and biofeedback, Delorme's perianal mucosal resection, laparoscopic or open surgical rectopexy ± sigmoid resection (rectum is 'hitched' up on to sacrum). Prolapse in young children is normally self-resolving and associated with straining.

Perianal haematoma

Very painful subcutaneous haematoma caused by rupture of small blood vessel in the perianal area. Evacuation of the clot provides instant relief.

Anal fissure

Definition

Longitudinal tear in the mucosa of the anal canal, in the midline posteriorly (90%) or anteriorly (10%).

Aetiology

- 90% caused by local trauma during passage of constipated stool and potentiated by spasm of the internal anal sphincter.
- Other causes: pregnancy/delivery, Crohn's disease, sexually transmitted infections (often lateral position).

Clinical features

Exquisitely painful on passing bowel motion, small amount of bright red blood on toilet tissue, severe sphincter spasm, skin tag at distal end of tear ('sentinel pile').

Treatment

- First-line: stool softeners/bulking agents, LA gels, 0.2/0.4% nitroglycerine ointment, topical calcium-channel blockers.

- Second-line: botulinum toxin injection (especially in women), lateral internal sphincterotomy (cures 95% but may result in minor incontinence in 10% of patients).
- EUA and biopsy for atypical/suspicious abnormal fissures.

Perianal abscess

Aetiology

Focus of infection starts in anal glands ('cryptoglandular sepsis') and spreads into perianal tissues to cause:

- Perianal abscess: adjacent to anal margin.
- Ischiorectal abscess: in ischiorectal fossa.
- Para-rectal abscess: above levator ani.

Recurrent abscesses are likely to be due to underlying fistula *in ano*.

Clinical features

Painful, red, tender, swollen mass ± fever, rigors, sweating, tachycardia.

Treatment

Incision and drainage, antibiotics.

Fistula *in ano*

Definition and aetiology

Abnormal communication between the perianal skin and the anal canal, established and persisting following drainage of a perianal abscess. May be associated with Crohn's disease (multiple fistulae), UC or TB.

- Low: below 50% of the EAS.
- High: crossing 50% or more of the EAS.

Clinical features

Chronic perianal discharge, external orifice of track with granulation tissue seen perianally.

Treatment

- Low: probing and laying open the track (fistulotomy).
- High: seton insertion, core removal of the fistula track.

Pilonidal sinus

Definition

A blind-ending track containing hairs in the skin of the natal cleft. *Pilus* = hair, *nidus* = nest.

Aetiology

Repetitive trauma to sacrococcygeal region promotes hair migration into the skin in natal cleft.

Clinical features

May present as: natal cleft abscess, discharging sinus in midline posterior to anal margin with hair protruding from orifice, natal cleft itch/pain. May occur on dorsum of hands between fingers in barbers or shepherds.

Treatment

Good personal hygiene. Incision and drainage of abscesses, excision of sinus network (primary closure requires asymmetrical closure with flattening of natal cleft).

50 Intestinal obstruction

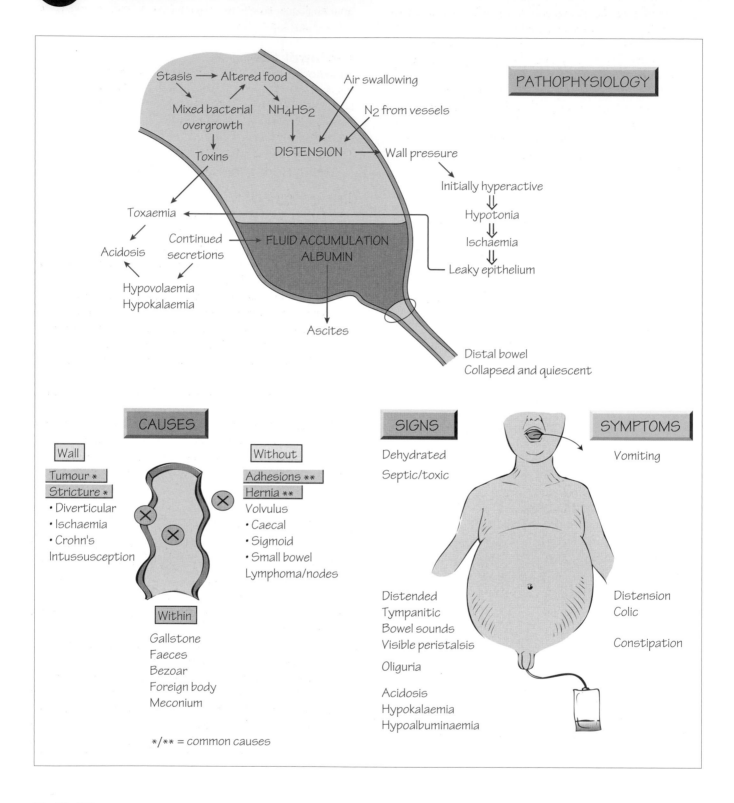

Definitions

Complete intestinal obstruction indicates total blockage of the intestinal lumen, whereas *incomplete* denotes only a partial blockage. Obstruction may be *acute* (hours) or *chronic* (weeks), *simple* (*mechanical*), i.e. blood supply is not compromised, or *strangulated*, i.e. blood supply is compromised. A *closed loop obstruction* indicates that both the inlet and outlet of a bowel loop is closed off. A *volvulus* is an abnormal twisting of a segment of the bowel causing intestinal obstruction and possible ischaemia and gangrene of the twisted segment.

 Surgery at a Glance, 4e. By P. Grace and N.R. Borley. Published 2009 by Blackwell Publishing. ISBN 978-1-4051-8325-3.

Common causes

- Extramural: adhesions, bands, volvulus, hernias (internal and external), compression by tumour (e.g. frozen pelvis).
- Intramural: inflammatory bowel disease (Crohn's disease), tumours, carcinomas, lymphomas, strictures, paralytic: (adynamic) ileus, intussusception.
- Intraluminal: faecal impaction, foreign bodies, bezoars, gallstone ileus.

Anatomical classification

Small bowel obstruction

Duodenum

- Adults: carcinoma of pancreas or periampullary carcinoma, chronic peptic ulcer disease.
- Neonates: duodenal atresia, annular pancreas, congential bands.

Jejunum/ileum

- Adults: adhesions, hernias, foreign body, tumours, Crohn's disease, Meckel's diverticulum.
- Neonates: meconium ileus, volvulus of malrotated gut, atresia, intussusception.

Large bowel obstruction

Colon

- Adults: tumours (usually left colon), diverticulitis, sigmoid volvulus, pseudo-obstruction.
- Neonates: Hirschsprung's disease, anal atresia.

Pathophysiology

- Bowel distal to obstruction collapses.
- Bowel proximal to obstruction distends and becomes hyperactive. Distension is due to swallowed air and accumulating intestinal secretions.
- The bowel wall becomes oedematous. Fluid and electrolytes accumulate in the wall and lumen (third space loss).
- Bacteria proliferate in the obstructed bowel.
- As the bowel distends, the intramural vessels become stretched and the blood supply is compromised, leading to ischaemia, necrosis and perforation.

Clinical features

- Vomiting, colicky abdominal pain, abdominal distension, absolute constipation (i.e. neither faeces nor flatus).
- Abdominal distension and increased bowel sounds.
- Dehydration and loss of skin turgor.
- Hypotension, tachycardia.
- Empty rectum on digital examination.
- Tenderness or rebound indicates peritonitis.

Investigations

- Hb, PCV: elevated due to dehydration.
- WCC: normal or slightly elevated.
- U+E: urea elevated, Na^+ and Cl^- low.
- Chest X-ray: elevated diaphragm due to abdominal distension.
- Abdominal supine X-ray:

  small bowel (central loops, non-anatomical distribution, valvulae conniventes shadows cross entire width of lumen like a ladder) or large bowel obstruction (peripheral distribution/haustral shadows do not cross entire width of bowel)

  look for cause (gallstone, characteristic patterns of volvulus, hernias)

  gas in the bowel wall (*pneumatosis intestinalis*) indicates gangene

- Single contrast large bowel enema—?large bowel obstruction—site and cause ('bird-beak' deformity with volvulus).
- Contrast CT scan—?small bowel obstruction—site and cause, colonoscopy/sigmoidoscopy to show site of obstruction.

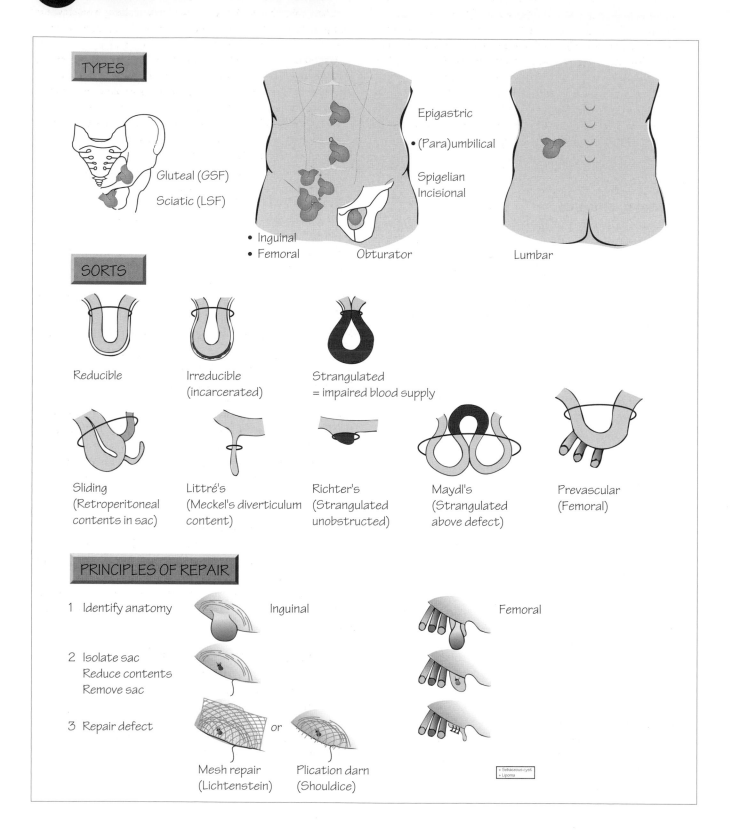

TYPES

Gluteal (GSF)

Sciatic (LSF)

Epigastric

• (Para)umbilical

Spigelian

Incisional

• Inguinal

• Femoral

Obturator

Lumbar

SORTS

Reducible

Irreducible
(incarcerated)

Strangulated
= impaired blood supply

Sliding
(Retroperitoneal
contents in sac)

Littré's
(Meckel's diverticulum
content)

Richter's
(Strangulated
unobstructed)

Maydl's
(Strangulated
above defect)

Prevascular
(Femoral)

PRINCIPLES OF REPAIR

1 Identify anatomy

Inguinal

Femoral

2 Isolate sac
    Reduce contents
    Remove sac

3 Repair defect

or

Mesh repair
(Lichtenstein)

Plication darn
(Shouldice)

+ Sebaceous cyst
+ Lipoma

Definitions

A *hernia* is the protrusion of a viscus or part of a viscus through an abnormal congenital or acquired opening in its coverings. An *abdominal wall hernia* is the protrusion of tissue (frequently peritoneum or fat) through an abnormal opening in the abdominal wall (frequently in the groin or umbilicus). The protruded peritoneum is the *hernial sac*. The *neck* of the hernia is the point where the sac passes through the defect in the abdominal wall and is often narrow. Sometimes a piece of intestine becomes trapped in the hernia (*incarcerated hernia*) and occasionally its blood supply is compromised (*strangulated hernia*).

Key points

- Abdominal wall hernias are common and cause many symptoms.
- Femoral hernias are more common in women than men but inguinal hernia is the most common hernia in women.
- All femoral hernias require prompt repair due to the risk of complications.
- Inguinal hernias may be repaired depending on symptoms.

Types

Common

- Umbilical/para-umbilical—common in adults and children.
- Inguinal (direct and indirect)—indirect common in infants.
- Femoral.
- Incisional.

Uncommon

- Epigastric.
- Spigelian, gluteal, lumbar, obturator.

Pathophysiology

- The defect in the abdominal wall may be congenital (e.g. umbilical hernia, femoral canal) or acquired (e.g. an incision) and is lined with peritoneum (the sac).
- Raised intra-abdominal pressure further weakens the defect allowing some of the intra-abdominal contents (e.g. omentum, small bowel loop) to migrate through the opening.
- Entrapment of the contents in the sac leads to incarceration (unable to reduce contents) and possibly strangulation (blood supply to incarcerated contents is compromised).

Clinical features

- Patient presents with a lump over the site of the hernia.
- Femoral hernias are below and lateral to the pubic tubercle, they usually flatten the groin crease and are 10 times more common in women than men. 50% present as a surgical emergency due to obstructed contents and 50% of these will require a small bowel resection. Femoral hernias are irreducible.
- Inguinal hernias start off above and medial to the pubic tubercle but may descend broadly when larger, they usually accentuate the groin crease. Most are benign and have a low risk of complications. Indirect inguinal hernias can be controlled by digital pressure over the internal inguinal ring, may be narrow-necked and are common in younger men (3% per annum present with complications). Direct inguinal hernias are poorly controlled by digital pressure, are often broad-necked and are more common in older men (0.3% per annum strangulate).
- Incisional hernias bulge, are usually broad-necked, poorly controlled by pressure and are accentuated by tensing the recti. Large, chronic, incisional hernias may contain much of the small bowel and may by irreducible/unrepairable due to the 'loss of the right of abode in the abdomen' of the contents.
- True umbilical hernias are present from birth and are symmetrical defects in the umbilicus. Most obliterate spontaneously by age 2. Only repair if persist after age 2–4 years.
- Para-umbilical hernias develop due to an acquired defect in the periumbilical fascia.

Essential management

- Assess the hernia for: severity of symptoms, risk of complications (type, size of neck), ease of repair (size, location), likelihood of success (size, loss of right of abode).
- Assess the patient for: fitness for surgery, impact of hernia on lifestyle (job, hobbies).
- Surgical repair is usually offered in suitable patients for:
  hernias at risk of complications whatever the symptoms
  hernias with previous symptoms of obstruction
  hernias at low risk of complications but symptoms interfering with lifestyle, etc.

Principles of hernia surgery

- Herniotomy: excision of the hernial sac alone for children.
- Herniorrhaphy: repairing the defect—mesh repair usual for inguinal hernias inserted via open or laparoscopic surgery.
- Incisional hernias may be repaired by open surgery or laparoscopically and usually require mesh to achieve satisfactory closure.

Complications of surgery

- Haematoma (wound or scrotal).
- Acute urinary retention.
- Wound infection.
- Chronic pain.
- Testicular pain and swelling leading to testicular atrophy.
- Hernia recurrence (about 2%).

	Causes and symptoms	Cardinal symptoms and signs	Structure involved (diagnosis)		
			Gallbladder	CBD	Other
A	Presence of stone → Irritation → Contraction	Pain Nausea Vomiting Tender RUQ	Biliary colic ↓ May	Biliary (ductal) colic ↓ May	—
B	Obstruction of structure (simple)	As above + • Persistence of pain etc. • Mass RUQ (jaundice)	Mucocele ↓ May	Obstructive jaundice ↓ May	—
C	Obstruction of structure (+ infection)	As above + • Swinging fever • Tachycardia • Neutrophilia • Rigors	Empyema ↓ May perforate Biliary peritonitis	Cholangitis	—
D	Inflammation/ infection	As for A + • Fever • Tachycardia • Neutrophilia	Cholecystitis	(Cholangitis)	Pancreatitis

Other conditions associated with gallstones
• Gallstone ileus
• Adenocarcinoma gallbladder

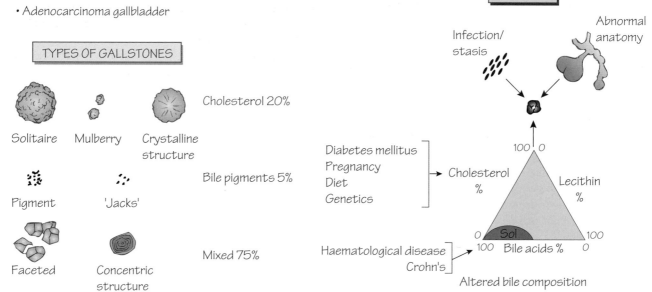

TYPES OF GALLSTONES

Solitaire   Mulberry   Crystalline structure   Cholesterol 20%

Pigment   'Jacks'   Bile pigments 5%

Faceted   Concentric structure   Mixed 75%

CAUSES

Infection/ stasis   Abnormal anatomy

Diabetes mellitus
Pregnancy   → Cholesterol %
Diet
Genetics

Haematological disease
Crohn's   → Bile acids %

Altered bile composition

Definition

Gallstones are round, oval or faceted concretions found in the biliary tract. They contain cholesterol, calcium carbonate, calcium bilirubinate or a mixture of these elements. Microlithiasis/microcrystalline disease is the presence of small/microscopic solid elements within the bile.

Key points

• Gallstones are common and not all causes of RUQ pain with an ultrasound scan showing stones are due to gallstones.
• One or more episodes of proven biliary colic may be managed by dietary and lifestyles measures and do not necessarily indicate cholecystectomy.
• An episode of obstructive jaundice, deranged LFTs or acute pancreatitis or a dilated common bile duct on ultrasound scan suggests the presence of common bile duct stones.
• A single attack of acute pancreatitis, cholangitis or obstructive jaundice is usually an indication for prophylactic cholecystectomy.

Epidemiology

Male : female 1 : 2. Age 40s onwards. High incidence of mixed stones in Western world. Pigment stones more common in the East.

Pathogenesis

• Cholesterol stones: imbalance in bile between cholesterol, bile salts and phospholipids, producing lithogenic bile. Associated with inflammatory bowel disease.
• Bilirubinate stones: chronic haemolysis, infection with glucuronidase-producing bacteria.
• Mixed stones: associated with anatomical abnormalities, stasis, previous surgery, previous infections.

Pathology

• Gallstones passing through the biliary system can cause biliary colic or pancreatitis.

• Stone obstruction at the gallbladder neck with superimposed infection leads to cholecystitis.
• Obstruction of the CBD with superimposed infection leads to septic cholangitis.
• Migration of a large stone into the gut may cause intestinal obstruction (gallstone ileus).

Clinical features

• 90% of gallstones are (probably) asymptomatic.
• Biliary colic: severe colicky upper abdominal pain radiating around the right costal margin ± vomiting. Periodicity of hours, often onset at night spontaneously resolves after several hours.

   Differential diagnosis includes myocardial infarction, peptic ulcer exacerbation, GORD.
• 'Chronic cholecystitis': uncertain diagnosis suggested by vague, intermittent, right upper abdominal pain, distension, flatulence, fatty food intolerance. May indicate recurrent mild episodes of cholecystitis. Differential diagnosis includes chronic PUD, GORD.
• Acute obstructive cholecystitis: constant right hypochondrial pain, pyrexia, nausea ± jaundice. Tender in RUQ with positive Murphy's sign. Leucocytosis. Unresolved may lead to an empyema of the gallbladder. Differential diagnosis includes myocardial infarction, basal pneumonia, pancreatitis, appendicitis, perforated peptic ulcer, pulmonary embolus.
• Cholangitis: abdominal pain, high fever/rigors, obstructive jaundice (Charcot's triad), severe RUQ tenderness. Differential diagnosis includes myocardial infarction, basal pneumonia, pancreatitis, acute hepatitis.
• Obstructive jaundice: upper abdominal pain, pale/claylike stools, dark brown urine, pruritus. May progress into cholangitis if CBD remains obstructed.
• Pancreatitis (see Chapter 53): central/epigastric pain, back pain, fever, tachycardia, epigastric tenderness.

Gallstone disease/2

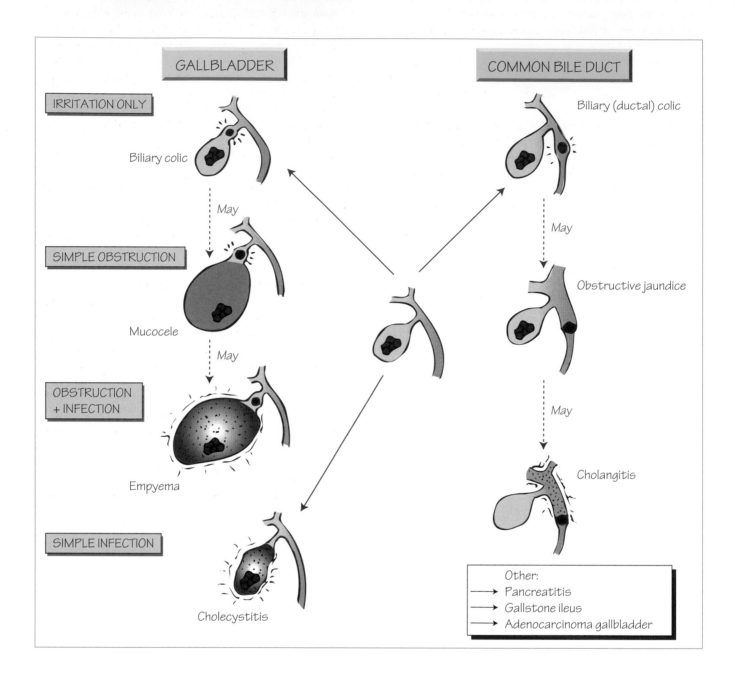

GALLBLADDER

IRRITATION ONLY

Biliary colic

May

SIMPLE OBSTRUCTION

Mucocele

May

OBSTRUCTION + INFECTION

Empyema

SIMPLE INFECTION

Cholecystitis

COMMON BILE DUCT

Biliary (ductal) colic

May

Obstructive jaundice

May

Cholangitis

Other:
→ Pancreatitis
→ Gallstone ileus
→ Adenocarcinoma gallbladder

Investigations

• FBC: acute inflammatory complications, picture of haemolytic anaemias underlying (microcytic anaemia).
• U+E: most important in jaundice to monitor renal function.
• LFTs: obstructive jaundice pattern.
• Plain X-ray of the abdomen shows only 10% of gallstones.
• Ultrasound: 90% of gallstones will be detected on ultrasound examination. Assesses CBD size and possible presence of CBD stones.
• MRCP is indicated for suspected CBD stones. If MRCP is positive then ERCP is indicated for CBD stone removal or stent placement.
• Endoluminal/transduodenal ultrasound—for the diagnosis of small ductal stones.
• OGD: to exclude PUD as a cause for uncomplicated disease symptoms.
• Rarely are other investigations required, such as oral cholecystography, intravenous cholangiography or HIDA scanning, especially where ultrasound is non-diagnostic, e.g. obesity).

Essential management

• Asymptomatic: no treatment required unless diabetic or undergoing major immunosuppression (risk factors for cholecystitis – prophylactic cholecystectomy may be indicated).
• Biliary colic: elective cholecystectomy, now usually performed laparoscopically, for classic symptoms with ultrasound-proven gallstones.
• Chronic cholecystitis: elective laparoscopic cholecystectomy only if no evidence of PUD or other causes for symptoms.
• Acute cholecystitis: IV fluids, antibiotics, early or interval cholecystectomy.
• Empyema: percutaneous (ultrasound- or CT-guided) drainage of the gallbladder and interval cholecystectomy.
• Ascending cholangitis: IV fluids, antibiotics, ductal drainage (now usually by ERCP, sphincterotomy and extraction of stones).

Complications of cholecystectomy

• Conversion—approximately 5–10% of laparoscopic cholecystectomies will have to be converted to an open operation (highest in males with previous inflammatory disease).
• Leakage of bile from cystic duct or gallbladder bed (Rx ERCP and temporary CBD stent, rarely percutaneous drainage).
• Jaundice due to retained ductal stones. (Retained stones can be treated by ERCP or if a T-tube is in place by extraction with a Dormia basket down the T-tube track (Burhenne manoeuvre).)
• Bleeding from cystic artery or gallbladder bed (may require re-operation).
• Injury to the CBD; usually requires major reconstructive surgery.

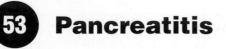

53 Pancreatitis

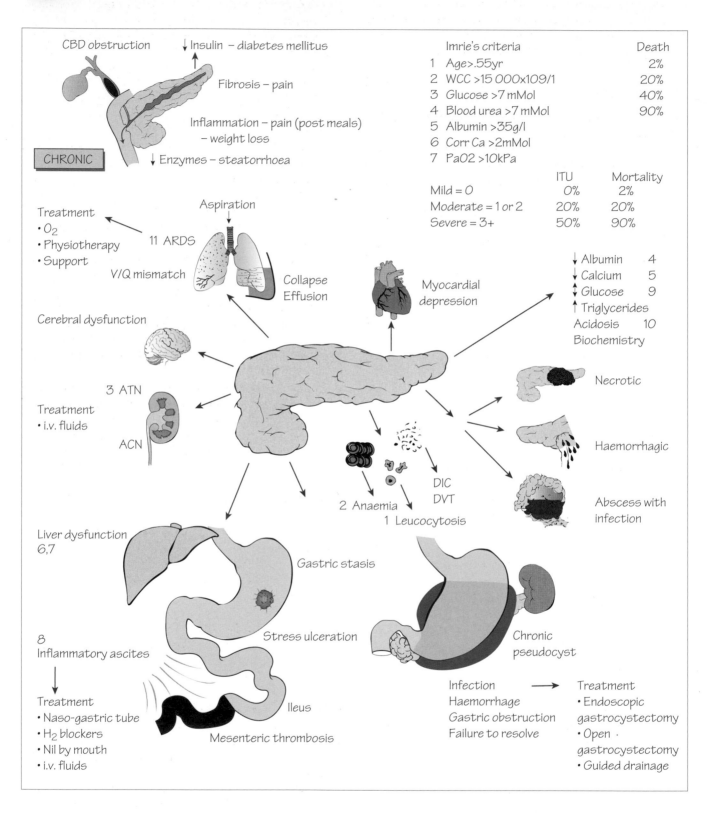

CBD obstruction

↓ Insulin – diabetes mellitus

Fibrosis – pain

Inflammation – pain (post meals)
– weight loss

CHRONIC

↓ Enzymes – steatorrhoea

Imrie's criteria		Death
1	Age>.55yr	2%
2	WCC >15 000x109/1	20%
3	Glucose >7 mMol	40%
4	Blood urea >7 mMol	90%
5	Albumin >35g/l	
6	Corr Ca >2mMol	
7	PaO2 >10kPa	

	ITU	Mortality
Mild = 0	0%	2%
Moderate = 1 or 2	20%	20%
Severe = 3+	50%	90%

Aspiration

Treatment
• O₂
• Physiotherapy
• Support

11 ARDS

V/Q mismatch

Collapse
Effusion

Myocardial
depression

↓ Albumin	4
↓ Calcium	5
↕ Glucose	9
↑ Triglycerides	
Acidosis	10
Biochemistry	

Cerebral dysfunction

3 ATN

Treatment
• i.v. fluids

ACN

Necrotic

Haemorrhagic

DIC
DVT

2 Anaemia

1 Leucocytosis

Abscess with
infection

Liver dysfunction
6,7

Gastric stasis

Stress ulceration

Chronic
pseudocyst

8
Inflammatory ascites

↓

Treatment
• Naso-gastric tube
• H₂ blockers
• Nil by mouth
• i.v. fluids

Ileus

Mesenteric thrombosis

Infection ⟶ Treatment
Haemorrhage
Gastric obstruction
Failure to resolve
• Endoscopic
gastrocystectomy
• Open
gastrocystectomy
• Guided drainage

Definition

Pancreatitis is an inflammatory condition of the exocrine pancreas that results from injury to the acinar cells. It may be acute or chronic. A *pancreatic pseudocyst* is a persisting accumulation of inflammatory fluid, usually in the lesser sac. It is called a *pseudo*cyst because it does not have an epithelial lining.

Key points

- Most pancreatitis (>80%) is mild and spontaneously resolves.
- All patients should have a cause sought by imaging and the severity assessed by recognized criteria.
- A normal or mildly elevated serum amylase does *not* exclude pancreatitis.
- Severe or complicated pancreatitis may worsen rapidly and require ICU support.
- Surgery has little place other than to treat severe complications.

Aetiology

- Gallstones and alcohol abuse account for 95% of cases of acute pancreatitis.
- Other causes include: Idiopathic, congenital structural abnormalities, drugs, viral infections, hypercalcaemia, hypothermia, hyperlipidaemia and trauma.

Pathology
Acute

- Mild injury: acinar (exocrine) cell damage with enzymatic spillage, inflammatory cascade activation and localized oedema. Local exudate may also lead to increased serum levels of pancreatic enzymes (amylase, lipase, colipase).
- Moderate injury: increasing local inflammation leads to intrapancreatic bleeding, fluid collections and spreading local oedema involving the mesentery and retroperitoneum. Activation of the systemic inflammatory response leads to progressive involvement of other organs.
- Severe injury: progressive pancreatic destruction leads to necrosis, profound localized bleeding and fluid collections around the pancreas. Spread to local structures and the peritoneal cavity may result in mesenteric infarction, peritonitis and intra-abdominal fat 'saponification'.

Chronic

Recurrent episodes of acute inflammation lead to progressive destruction of acinar cells with healing by fibrosis. Incidental islet cell damage may lead to endocrine gland failure.

Clinical features

- Mild/moderate pancreatitis: constant upper abdominal pain radiating to back, nausea, vomiting, pyrexia, tachycardia ± jaundice.
- Severe/necrotizing pancreatitis: severe upper abdominal pain, signs of hypovolaemic shock, respiratory and renal impairment, silent abdomen, retroperitoneal bleeding with flank and umbilical bruising (Grey Turner's and Cullen's signs).

Essential management

- Attempt to confirm diagnosis: (serum amylase >1000 iµ diagnostic—may be clinical diagnosis).
- Assess disease severity (Imrie criteria): severe is 3+ of the following:
  age >55 years
  WBC >15×10^9/L
  Pao_2 <10 kPa
  B glucose >7 mmol/L
  albumin <35 g/L
  urea >7 mmol/L
  Ca^{2+} <2.0 mmol/L.
- Resuscitate the patient:
  mild/moderate disease: IV fluids, analgesia, monitor progress with pulse, BP, temperature
  severe pancreatitis: full resuscitation in ICU with invasive monitoring
- Establish the cause: ultrasound to look for gallstones, CT to assess state of pancreas.

Further management

- No proven use for routine nasogastric tube or antibiotics.
- ?Vitamin supplements and sedatives if alcoholic cause.
- Proven CBD gallstones may require urgent ERCP and biliary drainage.
- Failure to respond to treatment or uncertain diagnosis warrants abdominal CT scan (the most reliable imaging modality in diagnosis of acute pancreatitis).
- Suspected/proven infection of necrotic pancreas—antibiotics ± surgical débridement.

Complications—acute pancreatitis
Acute

- Pancreatic abscess: usually necrotic pancreas present.
- Intra-abdominal sepsis.
- Necrosis of the transverse colon.
- Respiratory (ARDS) or renal (ATN) failure.
- Pancreatic haemorrhage.

Subacute/chronic

- Pseudocyst formation: may need to be drained internally or externally.
- Chronic pancreatitis.

Chronic pancreatitis

- Usually caused by chronic alcohol abuse.
- Presents with intractable abdominal pain and evidence of exocrine pancreatic failure (steatorrhoea) and eventually diabetes as well.
- Medical treatment is with analgesia and exocrine pancreatic enzyme replacement. Surgical treatment is by drainage of dilated pancreatic ducts or excision of the pancreas in some cases.

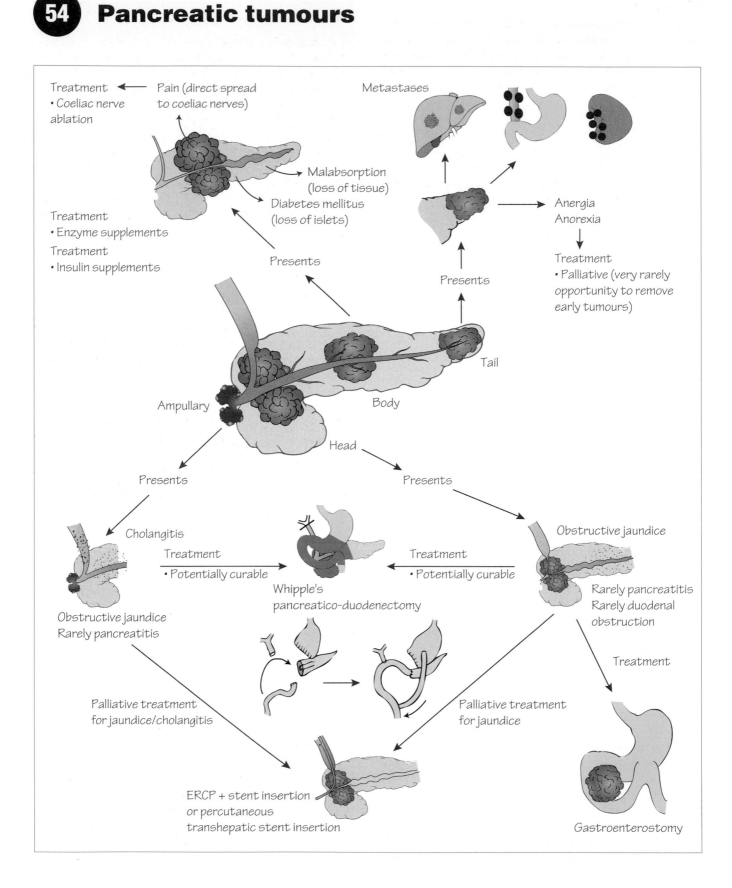

Treatment
• Coeliac nerve ablation

Pain (direct spread to coeliac nerves)

Metastases

Malabsorption (loss of tissue)
Diabetes mellitus (loss of islets)

Treatment
• Enzyme supplements
Treatment
• Insulin supplements

Presents

Anergia
Anorexia

Treatment
• Palliative (very rarely opportunity to remove early tumours)

Presents

Ampullary

Body

Tail

Head

Presents

Presents

Cholangitis

Treatment
• Potentially curable

Treatment
• Potentially curable

Obstructive jaundice

Obstructive jaundice
Rarely pancreatitis

Whipple's pancreatico-duodenectomy

Rarely pancreatitis
Rarely duodenal obstruction

Treatment

Palliative treatment for jaundice/cholangitis

Palliative treatment for jaundice

ERCP + stent insertion or percutaneous transhepatic stent insertion

Gastroenterostomy

Definitions

Pancreatic adenocarcinoma is a malignant lesion of the head, body or tail of the pancreas. *Periampullary carcinomas* arise around the ampulla of Vater and include tumours arising from the pancreas, duodenum, distal bile duct and the ampulla itself. *Endocrine pancreatic tumours* cause a variety of syndromes secondary to the secretion of active peptides.

Key points

- Most pancreatic cancer is not surgically curable.
- New, chronic back pain and vague symptoms may be the only presenting feature.
- The best prognosis is for true periampullary cancers.
- Good palliation of jaundice is possible without surgery.

Epidemiology

Male : female 2 : 1, peak incidence 50–70 years. Incidence of pancreatic carcinoma is increasing in the Western world.

Aetiology

Predisposing factors: smoking, diabetes, chronic pancreatitis.

Pathology

- Site: 55% involve head of pancreas, 25% body, 15% tail, 5% periampullary region.
- Macroscopic: growth is hard and infiltrating.
- Histology: 90% ductal carcinoma, 7% acinar cell carcinoma, 2% cystic carcinoma, 1% connective tissue origins.
- Spread:
  local into vital structures (portal vein, superior mesenteric vessels)
  lymphatics to peritoneum and regional nodes
  via bloodstream to liver and lung—metastases often present at time of diagnosis.

Clinical features

- Head or periampullary: painless, progressive jaundice with a palpable gallbladder (Courvoisier's law: a palpable gallbladder in the presence of jaundice is unlikely to be due to gallstones).
- Occasionally, duodenal obstruction causing vomiting.
- Body: back pain, anorexia, weight loss, steatorrhoea.
- Tail: often presents with metastases, malignant ascites or unexplained anaemia.

Investigations

- Ultrasound: may see mass in head of pancreas and distended biliary tree, facilitates needle biopsy.
- CT scan: demonstrates tumour mass, facilitates biopsy, assess involvement of surrounding structures and local lymph node spread.
- MRCP/ERCP: very accurate in making diagnosis; obtain specimen or shed cells for cytology and stent may be placed to relieve jaundice.
- Barium meal: widening of the duodenal loop with medial filling defect, the reversed '3' sign.

Essential management

Palliation

- Pancreatic adenocarcinoma is usually incurable at time of diagnosis.
- Jaundice can be relieved by placing a stent through the tumour either transhepatically or via ERCP/combined procedure.
- Duodenal obstruction may be relieved by gastrojejunostomy.
- Pain may be helped with a coeliac axis block.

Curative treatment

Rarely, surgical (Whipple's) resection of small tumours of the head of the pancreas is curative if lymph nodes are not involved.

Prognosis

- 90% of patients with pancreatic adenocarcinoma are dead within 12 months of diagnosis.
- It is important to obtain histology from tumours around the head of the pancreas as the prognosis from non-pancreatic periampullary cancers is considerably better (50% 5-year survival) following resection.

2 Week wait referral criteria for suspected upper GI cancer

- New-onset dysphagia (any age).
- Dyspepsia + weight loss/anaemia/vomiting.
- Dyspepsia + FHx/Barrett's oesophagus/previous peptic ulcer surgery/atrophic gastritis/pernicious anaemia.
- New dyspepsia >55 years.
- Jaundice.
- Upper abdominal mass.

Endocrine pancreatic tumours

- Rare (4–12 per million population), any age, male : female 1 : 1.
- Classified into non-functioning (50%) and functioning (insulinomas [25%], gastrinomas [15%], VIP-omas, glucagonomas and somatostatinomas [15%]).
- 15–30% of patients with pancreatic endocrine tumours have MEN type 1: (3 P's) parathyroid (hyperparathyroidism), pancreas (gastrinoma), pituitary (prolactinoma).
- Diagnosis:
  imaging: ultrasound, EUS, CT, MRI, MRA, SRS
  biochemistry: chromogranin A (general tumour marker increased in most endocrine tumours), hormone levels.
- Treatment: surgery, chemotherapy.
- Prognosis: 5-year survival: local disease 60–100%, regional disease 40%, distant metastases 30%.

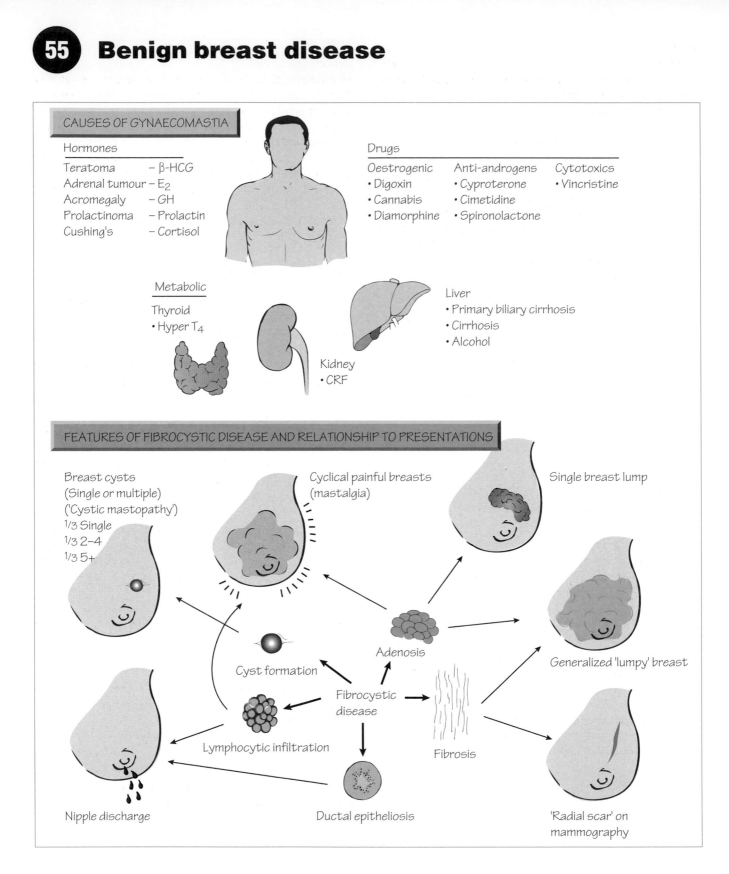

CAUSES OF GYNAECOMASTIA

Hormones

Teratoma	– β-HCG
Adrenal tumour	– E_2
Acromegaly	– GH
Prolactinoma	– Prolactin
Cushing's	– Cortisol

Drugs

Oestrogenic	Anti-androgens	Cytotoxics
• Digoxin	• Cyproterone	• Vincristine
• Cannabis	• Cimetidine	
• Diamorphine	• Spironolactone	

Metabolic

Thyroid
• Hyper T_4

Kidney
• CRF

Liver
• Primary biliary cirrhosis
• Cirrhosis
• Alcohol

FEATURES OF FIBROCYSTIC DISEASE AND RELATIONSHIP TO PRESENTATIONS

Breast cysts
(Single or multiple)
('Cystic mastopathy')
1/3 Single
1/3 2–4
1/3 5+

Cyclical painful breasts
(mastalgia)

Single breast lump

Cyst formation

Adenosis

Generalized 'lumpy' breast

Fibrocystic
disease

Fibrosis

Lymphocytic infiltration

Nipple discharge

Ductal epitheliosis

'Radial scar' on
mammography

ANDI

Definition

Abnormalities of the normal development and involution of the breast (ANDI)—a broad term covering benign conditions many of which have overlapping features.

> ### Key points
>
> • Any breast lump should be evaluated by triple assessment for risk of malignancy whatever the likely diagnosis.
> • Triple assessment is the combination of clinical examination, imaging (mammography for women aged 35 or over and ultrasonography for women aged under 35) and FNAC.
> • ANDI disorders are common in younger, premenopausal women and often cause considerable anxiety.
> • Gynaecomastia is usually physiological but often needs to be investigated for hormonal causes.

Abnormalities of development

Fibroadenoma

• Benign breast lump caused by overgrowth of single breast lobule. Manifests as one or more firm, mobile, painless lumps usually in women under 30 years.
• Investigation: 'triple assessment' (clinical/radiological/cytological).
• Treatment:
  age 30 years: either observe or excise if worried
  age 30 years: consider excision to exclude malignancy.

Abnormalities of cycles

Fibrocystic disease

• Usually presents age 25–45 years. May present as breast pain, tenderness, breast lump(s), breast cyst(s), especially during the second half of the menstrual cycle.
• Investigation: 'triple assessment' of all lumps.
• Treatment: patient reassurance, analgesics, γ-linoleic acid, hormone manipulation, cyst aspiration, excision of persistent localized masses after aspiration. Avoid xanthine-containing substances (coffee).

Abnormalities of involution

Breast cyst

• May be single or multiple. Firm, round, discrete lump(s).
• Investigation: aspiration ± mammography. Triple assessment for any discrete associated lumps.
• Treatment: reassurance, aspiration (repeated), hormone manipulation.

Other benign conditions

Breast abscess

• Usually infection of the pregnant or lactating breast with *Staphylococcus aureus* (puerperal infection). Patient presents with redness, swelling, heat and pain in the breast. Chronic/recurrent sepsis associated with smoking and ductal ectasia with mixed anaerobic infection.
• Treatment: puerperal sepsis is with antibiotics (flucloxacillin) initially but, if an abscess develops, repeated aspiration (or occasionally incision and drainage) will be required. Lactation/breastfeeding does not need to be suppressed while the abscess is being treated; treat chronic sepsis with metronidazole and recurrent aspirations if necessary.

Mammary duct ectasia

• Dilated subareolar ducts are filled with cellular debris which causes a periductal inflammatory response. Associated with smoking and recurrent non-lactational abscesses. The usual presentation is a green, multifocal, ductal nipple discharge and a subareolar lump.
• Treatment is by subareolar excision of the involved ducts if troublesome symptoms persist or the diagnosis is unsure.

Duct papilloma

• Small papillomas arise in the major breast ducts. They cause a bloody or serous nipple discharge usually from one duct.
• Treatment is usually by excision of the affected duct by microdochectomy if the symptoms persist.

Fat necrosis

• A fibrous scar in the breast tissue caused by injury, haematoma and necrosis of breast fat with subsequent scarring. History of trauma to the breast in 50% of cases. May be associated with superficial ecchymoses. Histology: periductal cellular infiltrate and fibrosis.
• Investigation: triple assessment.
• Treatment: surgical excision if mass fails to resolve or there is concern to exclude malignancy.

Cystosarcoma phylloides

• Large, predominantly benign (90%), fleshy, non-epithelial tumour of the breast presenting in middle age. Accounts for 1% of all breast tumours.
• Incisional or excisional biopsy is required to make a firm diagnosis.
• Wide local excision is the treatment of choice.
• Local recurrence is high with inadequate excision.
• Malignant lesions frequently metastasize to the lungs—prognosis is poor.

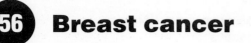

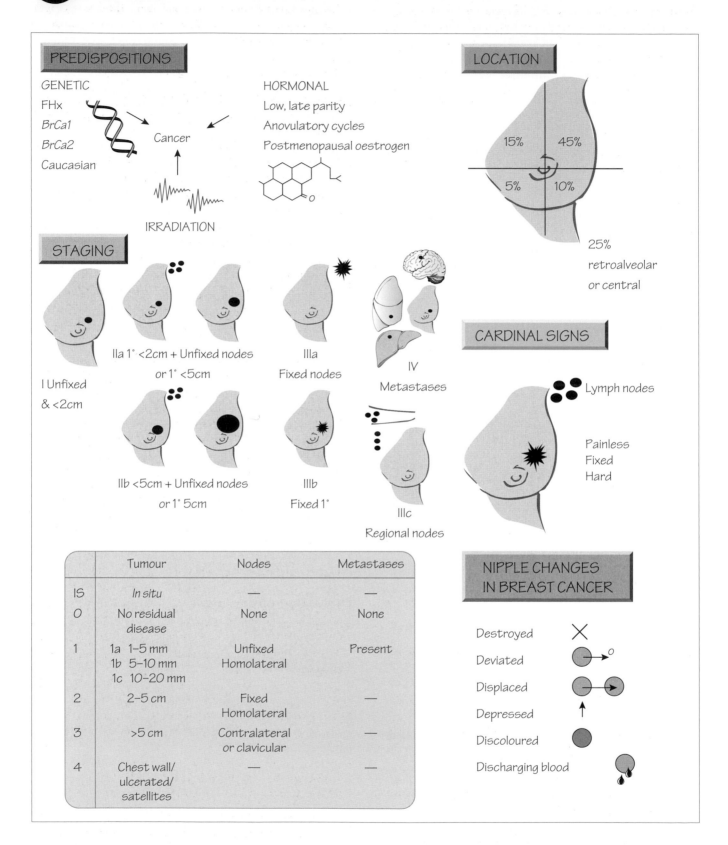

PREDISPOSITIONS

GENETIC
FHx
BrCa1
BrCa2
Caucasian

Cancer

IRRADIATION

HORMONAL
Low, late parity
Anovulatory cycles
Postmenopausal oestrogen

LOCATION

15%   45%

5%   10%

25% retroalveolar or central

STAGING

I Unfixed & <2cm

IIa 1° <2cm + Unfixed nodes or 1° <5cm

IIIa Fixed nodes

IV Metastases

IIb <5cm + Unfixed nodes or 1° 5cm

IIIb Fixed 1°

IIIc Regional nodes

CARDINAL SIGNS

Lymph nodes

Painless
Fixed
Hard

	Tumour	Nodes	Metastases
IS	*In situ*	—	—
0	No residual disease	None	None
1	1a 1–5 mm 1b 5–10 mm 1c 10–20 mm	Unfixed Homolateral	Present
2	2–5 cm	Fixed Homolateral	—
3	>5 cm	Contralateral or clavicular	—
4	Chest wall/ ulcerated/ satellites	—	—

NIPPLE CHANGES IN BREAST CANCER

Destroyed

Deviated

Displaced

Depressed

Discoloured

Discharging blood

Definition

Malignant lesion of (predominantly) the female breast.

Epidemiology

Male : female 1 : 100. Usually >30 years. One in nine women will develop breast cancer in their lifetime.

Aetiology

- Strong family history of breast cancer (genetic factors— BRCA1 or BRCA2 mutated gene).
- High premenopausal blood IGF-1 level.
- Early menarche and late menopause, especially in nulliparous women.
- Social class I and II.

Pathology

- Histology: adenocarcinomas (glandular epithelium). Common types are invasive ductal (90%) or lobular (10%) carcinoma. Paget's disease is ductal carcinoma involving the nipple.
- Spread: lymphatics, direct extension; haematogenous to lung, liver, bone, brain, adrenal, ovary.
- Staging: TNM classification—important for treatment and prognosis. Also Stages I, IIA, IIB, IIIA, IIIB and IV.

Screening

- Women aged 50–70 years should be screened for breast cancer every 3 years by two-view (craniocaudal and mediolateral) mammography.
- Participation in national screening programmes reduces breast cancer mortality by 35%.

Clinical features

- Palpable, hard, irregular, fixed breast lump, usually painless.
- Nipple retraction and skin dimpling.
- Nipple eczema in Paget's disease.
- Peau d'orange (cutaneous oedema 2° lymphatic obstruction).
- Palpable axillary nodes.

Investigations

- Triple assessment: clinical examination/imaging/cytology.
- Imaging: mammography: irregular, spiculated, radio-opaque mass with microcalcification. Not used under age 35 years unless strong clinical suspicion of carcinoma.
   ultrasound: women <35 years with dense or large breasts.
   MRI: helpful when U/S not diagnostic. Indicated for axillary disease without obvious primary source.
- Cytological assessment: FNAC or core biopsy.
- Breast biopsy: excision biopsy occasionally required for diagnosis.
- Staging investigations for proven carcinoma: all: CXR, FBC, serum alkaline phosphatase, γ-GT and calcium only if metatsases clinically suspected: isotope bone scan, U/S liver, brain CT scan.
- Breast tissue for hormone receptor status (ER + or −, progesterone receptor + or −, HER2/neuHuman + or −) important for treatment and prognosis.

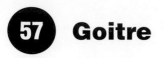

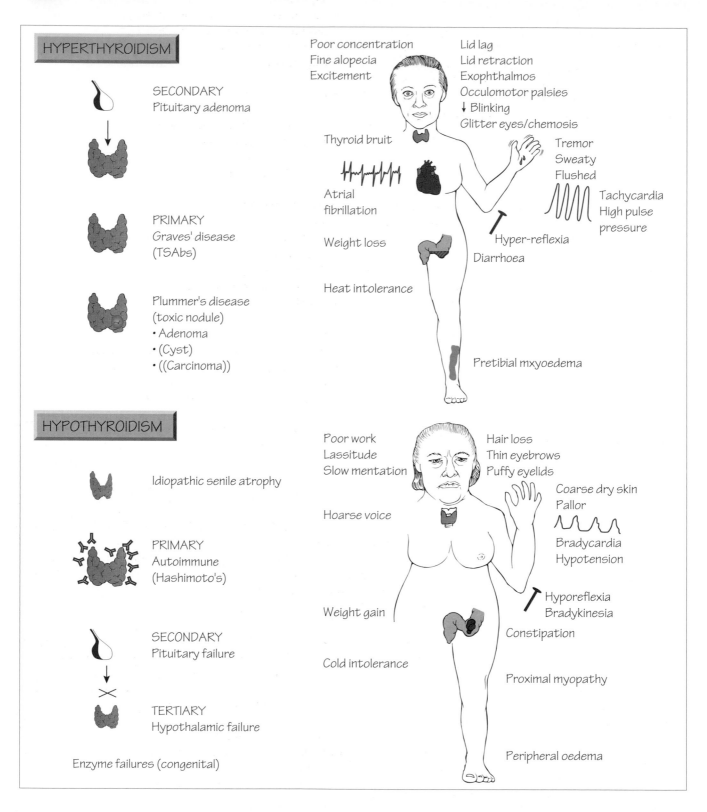

HYPERTHYROIDISM

SECONDARY
Pituitary adenoma

PRIMARY
Graves' disease
(TSAbs)

Plummer's disease
(toxic nodule)
• Adenoma
• (Cyst)
• ((Carcinoma))

Poor concentration
Fine alopecia
Excitement

Lid lag
Lid retraction
Exophthalmos
Occulomotor palsies
↓ Blinking
Glitter eyes/chemosis

Thyroid bruit

Atrial
fibrillation

Weight loss

Heat intolerance

Tremor
Sweaty
Flushed

Tachycardia
High pulse
pressure

Hyper-reflexia

Diarrhoea

Pretibial mxyoedema

HYPOTHYROIDISM

Idiopathic senile atrophy

PRIMARY
Autoimmune
(Hashimoto's)

SECONDARY
Pituitary failure

TERTIARY
Hypothalamic failure

Enzyme failures (congenital)

Poor work
Lassitude
Slow mentation

Hair loss
Thin eyebrows
Puffy eyelids

Hoarse voice

Coarse dry skin
Pallor

Bradycardia
Hypotension

Hyporeflexia
Bradykinesia

Weight gain

Constipation

Cold intolerance

Proximal myopathy

Peripheral oedema

134 *Surgery at a Glance*, 4e. By P. Grace and N.R. Borley. Published 2009 by Blackwell Publishing. ISBN 978-1-4051-8325-3.

Definition

A *goitre* is an enlargement of the thyroid gland from any cause.

Key points

- Toxic goitres are rarely malignant.
- All solitary nodules need investigation (U/S, radionuclide imaging, FNAC) to exclude carcinoma.
- Surgery is rarely necessary in autoimmune or inflammatory thyroid disease.

Common causes

- Physiological: gland increases in size as a result of increased demand for thyroid hormone at puberty and during pregnancy.
- Iodine deficiency (endemic): deficiency of iodine results in decreased T_4 levels and increased TSH stimulation leading to a diffuse goitre.
- Primary hyperthyroidism (Graves' disease): goitre and thyrotoxicosis due to circulating immunoglobulin LATS.
- Adenomatous (nodular) goitre: benign hyperplasia of the thyroid gland.
- Thyroiditis: autoimmune (Hashimoto's); subacute (de Quervain's); Riedel's (struma).
- Thyroid malignancies.

Clinical features

Hyperthyroidism

Symptoms

- Heat intolerance and excessive sweating.
- Increased appetite, weight loss, diarrhoea.
- Anxiety, tiredness, palpitations.
- Oligomenorrhoea.

Signs

- Goitre.
- Exophthalmos, lid lag and retraction.
- Warm moist palms, tremor.
- Atrial fibrillation.
- Pretibial myxoedema.

Hypothyroidism

Symptoms

- Cold intolerance, decreased sweating.
- Hoarseness.
- Weight increase, constipation.
- Slow cerebration, tiredness.
- Muscle pains.

Signs

- Pale/yellow skin, dry, thickened skin, thin hair.
- Periorbital puffiness, loss of outer third of eyebrow.
- Dementia, nerve deafness, hyporeflexia.
- Slow pulse, large tongue, peripheral oedema.

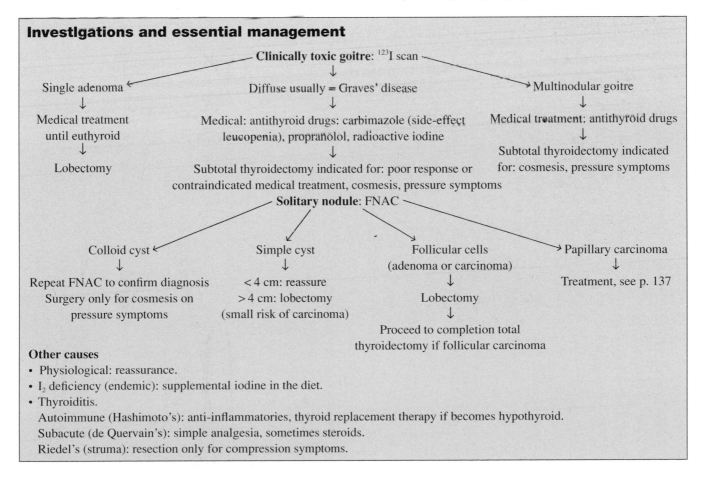

Investigations and essential management

Clinically toxic goitre: ^{123}I scan

Single adenoma → Medical treatment until euthyroid → Lobectomy

Diffuse usually = Graves' disease → Medical: antithyroid drugs: carbimazole (side-effect leucopenia), propranolol, radioactive iodine → Subtotal thyroidectomy indicated for: poor response or contraindicated medical treatment, cosmesis, pressure symptoms

Multinodular goitre → Medical treatment: antithyroid drugs → Subtotal thyroidectomy indicated for: cosmesis, pressure symptoms

Solitary nodule: FNAC

Colloid cyst → Repeat FNAC to confirm diagnosis. Surgery only for cosmesis on pressure symptoms

Simple cyst → < 4 cm: reassure. > 4 cm: lobectomy (small risk of carcinoma)

Follicular cells (adenoma or carcinoma) → Lobectomy → Proceed to completion total thyroidectomy if follicular carcinoma

Papillary carcinoma → Treatment, see p. 137

Other causes

- Physiological: reassurance.
- I_2 deficiency (endemic): supplemental iodine in the diet.
- Thyroiditis.
  Autoimmune (Hashimoto's): anti-inflammatories, thyroid replacement therapy if becomes hypothyroid.
  Subacute (de Quervain's): simple analgesia, sometimes steroids.
  Riedel's (struma): resection only for compression symptoms.

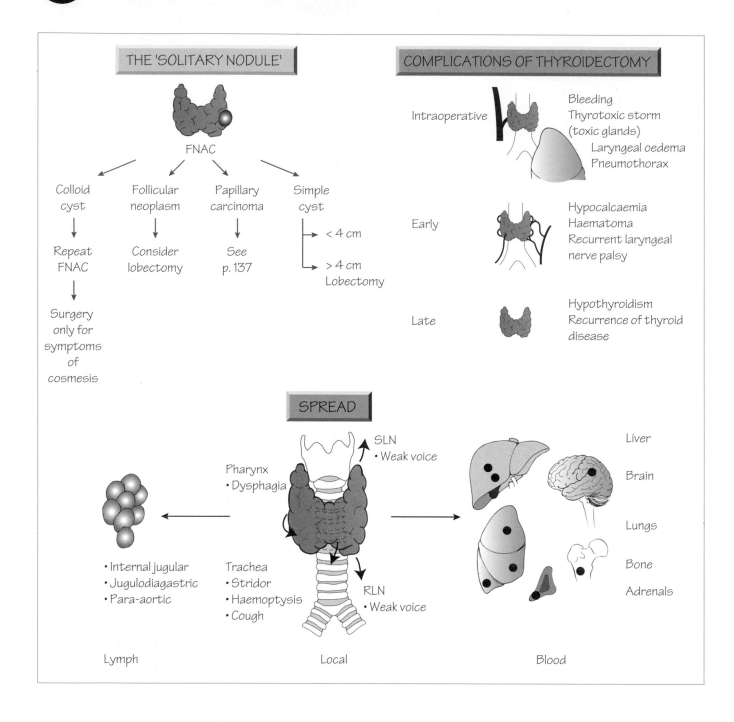

THE 'SOLITARY NODULE'

FNAC

- Colloid cyst → Repeat FNAC → Surgery only for symptoms of cosmesis
- Follicular neoplasm → Consider lobectomy
- Papillary carcinoma → See p. 137
- Simple cyst → < 4 cm / > 4 cm Lobectomy

COMPLICATIONS OF THYROIDECTOMY

Intraoperative
- Bleeding
- Thyrotoxic storm (toxic glands)
- Laryngeal oedema
- Pneumothorax

Early
- Hypocalcaemia
- Haematoma
- Recurrent laryngeal nerve palsy

Late
- Hypothyroidism
- Recurrence of thyroid disease

SPREAD

Lymph
- Internal jugular
- Jugulodiagastric
- Para-aortic

Local
- Pharynx
  - Dysphagia
- Trachea
  - Stridor
  - Haemoptysis
  - Cough
- SLN
  - Weak voice
- RLN
  - Weak voice

Blood
- Liver
- Brain
- Lungs
- Bone
- Adrenals

Definition
Malignant lesions of the thyroid gland.

Key points
- Many thyroid tumours are tumours of young adults. Occasionally occurs in childhood.
- Isolated thyroid lumps should always be investigated to confirm a cause.
- The prognosis is often good with surgical resection and medical adjuvant treatment.
- All patients should be managed by an MDT.

Epidemiology

Male : female 1 : 2. Peak incidence depends on histology (papillary, young adults; follicular, middle age; anaplastic, elderly; medullary, any age).

Pathology

Histology of thyroid malignancies.

Type	(% of total)	Cell of origin	Differentiation	Spread
Papillary	(60%)	Epithelial	Well	Lymphatic
Follicular	(25%)	Epithelial	Well	Haematogenous
Anaplastic	(10%)	Epithelial	Poor	Direct, lymphatic and haematogenous
Medullary	(5%)	Parafollicular	Moderate	Lymphatic and haematogenous

Aetiology

Predisposing factors:
  pre-existing goitre
  radiation of the neck in childhood.

Clinical features

- Papillary: solitary thyroid nodule.
- Follicular: slow-growing thyroid mass, symptoms from distant metastases.
- Anaplastic: rapidly growing thyroid mass causing tracheal and oesophageal compression.
- Medullary: thyroid lump, may have MEN IIA (medullary thyroid carcinoma, phaeochromocytoma, hyperparathyroidism) or MEN IIB (medullary thyroid carcinoma, phaeochromocytoma, multiple mucosal neuromas, Marfanoid habitus) syndrome.

Essential management

Papillary
- Surgery: total thyroidectomy and removal of involved lymph nodes.
- Adjunctive treatment: [131]I ablation and TSH suppression (T_4 therapy) (rationale: TSH production stimulates papillary tumour growth).
- Prognosis: excellent.

Follicular
- Surgery: thyroid lobectomy and removal of involved nodes for tumours <1 cm or total thyroidectomy and removal of involved nodes for tumours >1 cm or if metastases or local spread are present.
- Adjunctive treatment: TSH suppression (T_4 therapy) for all tumours. [131]I ablation and TSH suppression for tumours treated by total thyroidectomy.
- Prognosis: no metastases, 90% 10-year survival; metastases, 30% 10-year survival.

Anaplastic
- Surgery: only to relieve pressure symptoms.
- Adjunctive treatment: neither radiotherapy nor chemotherapy is effective.
- Prognosis: dismal—most patients will be dead within 12 months of diagnosis.

Medullary
- Exclude phaeochromocytoma before treating.
- Surgery: total thyroidectomy and excision of regional lymph nodes.
- Adjuvant radiotherapy and chemotherapy ineffective.
- Prognosis: overall 50% 5-year survival.

Investigations

- Ultrasound of the thyroid gland.
- FNAC: may give histological diagnosis.
- Bone scan and radiographs of bones for secondary deposits.
- Calcitonin levels as a marker for medullary carcinoma.
- Serum thyroglobulin is an excellent tumour marker in patients who have had total thyroidectomy and ^{131}I ablation.

Complications of thyroid surgery

- Postoperative bleeding: an expanding haematoma can cause laryngeal oedema and airway obstruction. Rx—relieve haematoma, intubate.
- Voice dysfunction: damage to recurrent or external laryngeal nerves (only 1% have permanent injury and few require treatment). Vocal cords should checked by laryngoscopy preoperatively.
- Hypocalcaemia: damage to parathyroid glands. Rx—500 mg elemental calcium t.d.s. ± vitamin D (alfacalcidol or calcitrol). If severe symptoms give calcium gluconate IV slowly.
- Hypothyroidism: expected consequence of total thyroidectomy. Measure TSH levels and replace with T_4 (or T_3).
- Thyrotoxic storm: rare now. May occur during or after surgery for Graves' disease. Rx—beta-blockade, steroids, iodine and propylthiouracil.

2 Week wait referral criteria for suspected head and neck cancer

- Horseness >6 weeks.
- Oral ulceration >3 weeks.
- Oral swellings >3 weeks.
- Dysphagia >3 weeks.
- Neck mass >3 weeks.
- Cranial neuropathies.
- Rapidly developed thyroid lump.

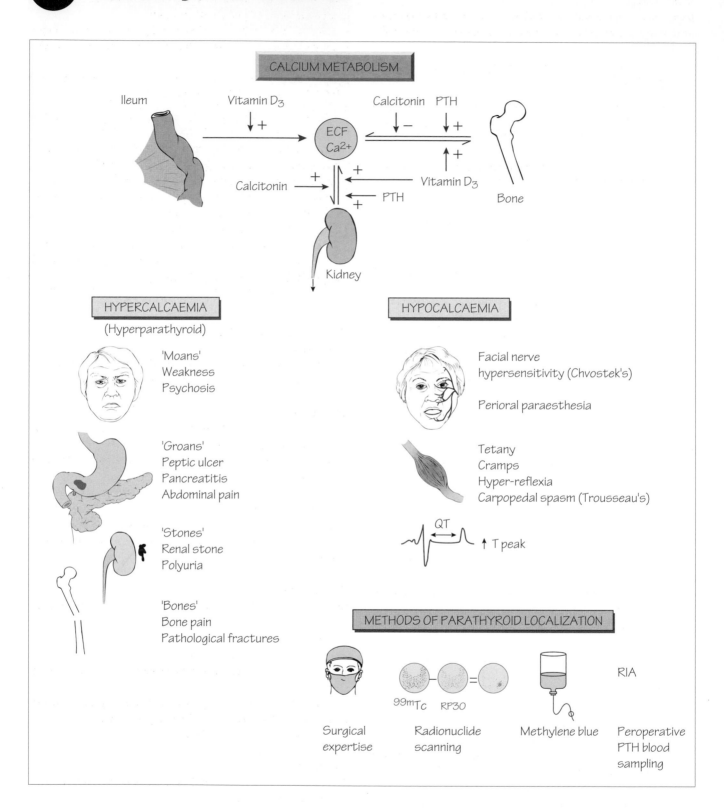

CALCIUM METABOLISM

Ileum Vitamin D₃ Calcitonin PTH

ECF Ca²⁺

Calcitonin Vitamin D₃ PTH

Kidney Bone

HYPERCALCAEMIA

(Hyperparathyroid)

'Moans'
Weakness
Psychosis

'Groans'
Peptic ulcer
Pancreatitis
Abdominal pain

'Stones'
Renal stone
Polyuria

'Bones'
Bone pain
Pathological fractures

HYPOCALCAEMIA

Facial nerve
hypersensitivity (Chvostek's)

Perioral paraesthesia

Tetany
Cramps
Hyper-reflexia
Carpopedal spasm (Trousseau's)

QT ↑ T peak

METHODS OF PARATHYROID LOCALIZATION

99mTc RP30 RIA

Surgical
expertise

Radionuclide
scanning

Methylene blue

Peroperative
PTH blood
sampling

Hyperparathyroidism

Definition

Hyperparathyroidism is a condition characterized by hypercalcaemia caused by excess production of parathyroid hormone (PTH).

> ### Key points
>
> - Hyperparathyroidism often presents with vague symptoms to many different specialists.
> - Surgery is the treatment of choice for primary hyperparathyroidism.
> - Hypoparathyroidism postsurgery is rare and mostly transient.

Causes

- *Primary* hyperparathyroidism is usually due to a parathyroid benign adenoma (75%) or parathyroid hyperplasia (20%). <0.5% have parathyroid carcinoma.
- *Secondary* hyperparathyroidism is hyperplasia of the gland in response to hypocalcaemia (e.g. in chronic renal failure).
- In *tertiary* hyperparathyroidism, autonomous secretion of parathormone occurs when the secondary stimulus has been removed (e.g. after renal transplantation).
- *MEN syndromes* (type I [parathyroid adenoma, pancreatic islet cell tumours, pituitary adenoma] and type II [parathyroid adenoma, medullary thyroid cancer, phaeochromocytoma) and *ectopic* parathormone production (e.g. oat cell carcinoma of the lung).

Pathology

Parathormone mobilizes calcium from bone, enhances renal tubular absorption and, with vitamin D, intestinal absorption of calcium. The net result is *hypercalcaemia*.

Clinical features

- Older women, >40 years of age.
- Renal calculi or renal calcification—occurs in 20% of patients, polyuria ('renal stones').
- Bone pain or deformity, osteitis fibrosa cystica, pathological fractures ('painful bones').
- Muscle weakness, anorexia, intestinal atony, psychosis ('psychic moans').
- Peptic ulceration and pancreatitis ('abdominal groans').

Diagnosis

Laboratory

- Elevated PTH in the setting of hypercalcaemia.
- Serum calcium (specimen taken on three occasions with patient fasting, at rest and without a tourniquet). Normal range 2.2–2.6 mmol/L. Calcium is bound to albumin and the level has to be 'corrected' when albumin levels are abnormal.
- May be decreased serum phosphate and elevated alkaline phosphatase.

Imaging

- High-resolution ultrasound.
- Dual isotope imaging using ^{99m}Tc sestamibi imaging.
- CT and MRI scanning.
- DXA scans for bone density measurement should be obtained in all patients with hyperparathyroidism.
- Selective vein catheterization and digital subtraction angiography in patients in whom exploration has been unsuccessful.

> ### Essential management
>
> - Treat hypercalcaemia if calcium levels very high (>2.88 mmol/L).
> - Primary and tertiary hyperparathyroidism are treated surgically: excise adenoma if present, remove 3.5 of 4 glands for hyperplasia. Intraoperative rapid PTH assay facilitates minimally invasive parathyroidectomy under LA with >95% success rate, i.e. return to normocalcaemia.
> - Secondary hyperplasia: vitamin D and/or calcium.
> - Cinacalcet, a calcimimetic drug that reduces PTH secretion and is indicated in patients with high PTH levels that cannot be lowered by other treatments.

Hypoparathyroidism

Definition

Hypoparathyroidism is a rare condition characterized by hypocalcaemia due to reduced production of parathormone.

Causes

- Post-thyroid or parathyroid surgery ('hungry bone syndrome') or neck irradiation.
- Idiopathic (often autoimmune and presents in children or young adults).
- Congenital enzymatic deficiencies (numerous syndromes).
- Metal overload (e.g. iron [haemochromatosis or thalassaemia], copper [Wilson's disease], magnesium).
- Pseudohypoparathyroidism (reduced sensitivity to parathormone).

Pathology

Reduced serum calcium increases neuromuscular excitability.

Clinical features

- Perioral paraesthesia, cramps, tetany.
- *Chvostek's sign*: tapping over facial nerve induces facial muscle contractions.
- *Trousseau's sign*: inflating BP cuff to above systolic pressure induces typical *main d'accoucheur* carpal spasm.
- Prolonged QT interval on ECG.

Diagnosis

Calcium and parathormone levels decreased. Also measure vitamin D and magnesium.

> ### Essential management
>
> Calcium and vitamin D.

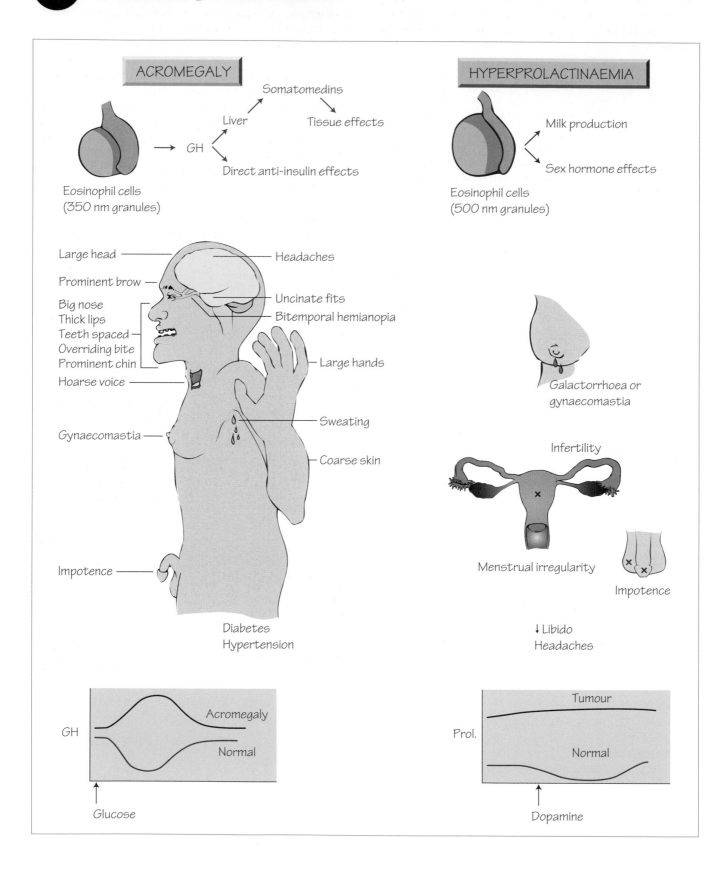

ACROMEGALY

Eosinophil cells
(350 nm granules)

GH → Liver → Somatomedins → Tissue effects

GH → Direct anti-insulin effects

Large head — Headaches
Prominent brow
Big nose
Thick lips
Teeth spaced — Uncinate fits
Overriding bite — Bitemporal hemianopia
Prominent chin
Hoarse voice — Large hands
Gynaecomastia — Sweating
Impotence — Coarse skin

Diabetes
Hypertension

GH   Acromegaly
      Normal
↑
Glucose

HYPERPROLACTINAEMIA

Eosinophil cells
(500 nm granules)

→ Milk production
→ Sex hormone effects

Galactorrhoea or
gynaecomastia

Infertility

Menstrual irregularity

Impotence

↓ Libido
Headaches

Prol.   Tumour
         Normal
↑
Dopamine

Definition

Pituitary disorders are characterized either by a *failure of secretion* of pituitary hormones or by tumours, which cause *local pressure effects* or specific syndromes due to *hormone overproduction.*

Key points

• Acromegaly is often insidious in onset and slow to be diagnosed.
• Deficiencies of pituitary function are generally tested for by stimulation tests and overactivity by suppressions tests. Occasionally, direct serum hormone levels may be measured.

Common causes

• Primary failure of *anterior* pituitary secretion (GH, gonadotrophins, TSH and ACTH) causes pan-hypopituitarism (Simmonds' disease):
  pressure from a tumour—adenoma or craniopharyngioma
  infarction or ischaemia—haemorrhagic shock, especially postpartum (Sheehan's syndrome)
  inflammatory—meningitis, pituitary abscess, sarcoidosis
  infiltrative—haemochromatosis
  iatrogenic—surgery, radiotherapy
• Secondary *anterior* pituitary secretion failure from hypothalamic causes.
• Failure of ADH production from the *posterior* pituitary gland leads to CDI. NDI results from renal resistance to ADH. Causes of CDI are:
  idiopathic—some genetic (abnormality of ADH gene on chromosome 20)
  trauma—especially skull base fractures
  tumours—sellar and suprasellar, e.g. craniopharyngioma
  granulomas—TB or sarcoidosis
  vascular—aneurysm or thrombosis

Clinical features

• Pan-hypopituitarism: pallor (MSH), hypothyroidism (TSH), failure of lactation (PL), chronic adrenal insufficiency (ACTH), delayed puberty, ovarian failure and amenorrhoea (FSH, LH). GH loss in adults is usually asymptomatic or may lead to loss of energy.

• Diabetes insipidus (ADH): insidious or abrupt onset of *polyuria* (5–20 L/day) and *polydipsia.*
• Tumours: clinical features of a mass lesion: (headache, bitemporal hemianopia, altered appetite, thirst).
• Hyperpituitarism is virtually always selective:
  acromegaly/gigantism (excess GH): thickened skin, increased skull size, prognathism, enlarged tongue, goitre, osteoporosis, organomegaly, spade-like hands and feet
  Cushing's disease (excess ACTH): malaise, muscle weakness, weight gain, bruising, moon facies, buffalo hump, hirsutism, amenorrhoea, impotence, polyuria, diabetes, emotional instability
  galactorrhoea (excess PL): spontaneous flow of milk from the nipple at any time other than during breastfeeding

Investigations

• Pan-hypopituitarism: serum assay of pituitary and target gland hormones, dynamic tests of pituitary function.
• CDI: very low urinary specific gravity (<1.005 and osmolality <200 mOsm/L) which does not increase with a *water deprivation test.*
• Tumours: visual field measurements, hormone assay, CT or MRI scanning.

Essential management

• Pan-hypopituitarism: replacement therapy—cyclical oestrogen—progesterone, hydrocortisone, thyroxine.
• Diabetes insipidus: vasopressin analogue, desmopressin, administered as nasal spray.
• Tumours: bromocriptine suppresses PL release from prolactinomas, ^{90}Y implant for pituitary ablation, surgery (hypophysectomy via nasal or transcranial route).

Tumours (% of total)	Cell type
Endocrinologically active (75%)	
Prolactinomas (35%)	Acidophil
GH-secreting tumours (20%)	Acidophil
Mixed PL and GH (10%)	Acidophil
ACTH-secreting tumours (10%)	Basophil
Endocrinologically inactive (25%)	Chromophobe
Craniopharyngioma	Rathke's pouch

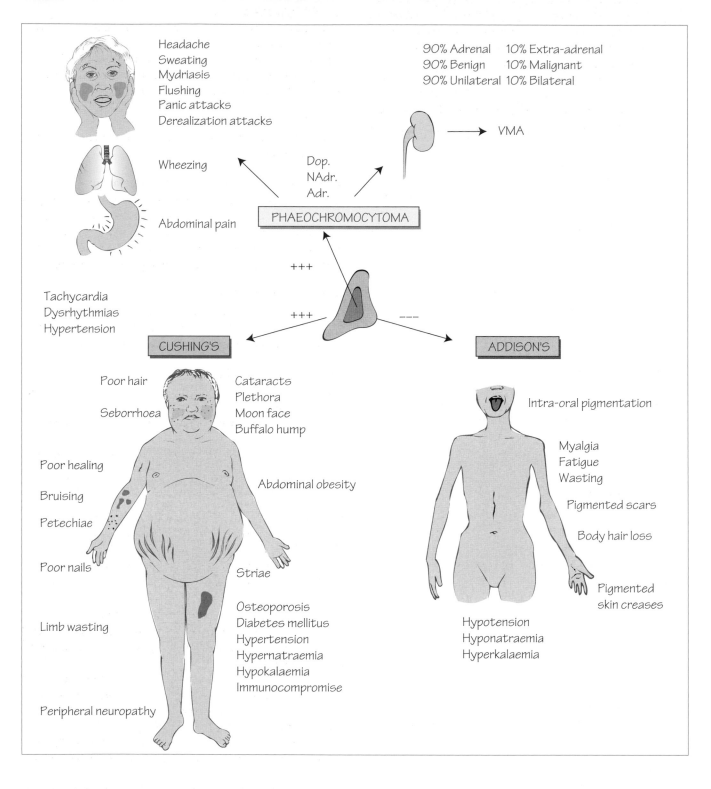

Headache
Sweating
Mydriasis
Flushing
Panic attacks
Derealization attacks

90% Adrenal   10% Extra-adrenal
90% Benign   10% Malignant
90% Unilateral 10% Bilateral

→ VMA

Wheezing

Dop.
NAdr.
Adr.

PHAEOCHROMOCYTOMA

Abdominal pain

+++

Tachycardia
Dysrhythmias
Hypertension

+++   ---

CUSHING'S   ADDISON'S

Poor hair

Cataracts
Plethora
Moon face
Buffalo hump

Intra-oral pigmentation

Seborrhoea

Myalgia
Fatigue
Wasting

Poor healing

Pigmented scars

Abdominal obesity

Bruising

Body hair loss

Petechiae

Poor nails

Pigmented
skin creases

Striae

Limb wasting

Osteoporosis
Diabetes mellitus
Hypertension
Hypernatraemia
Hypokalaemia
Immunocompromise

Hypotension
Hyponatraemia
Hyperkalaemia

Peripheral neuropathy

Definitions

Adrenal gland disorders are characterized by clinical syndromes resulting from either a *failure of secretion* or *excessive secretion* of adrenal cortical hormones (glucocorticoids [cortisol], mineralocorticoids [aldosterone], and androgens ([DHEA]) or medullary hormones (mostly adrenaline [epinephrine]). *Cushing's syndrome* describes the clinical features irrespective of the cause; *Cushing's disease* refers to a pituitary adenoma with secondary adrenal hyperplasia.

Common causes

Failure of secretion

Addison's disease or adrenal insufficiency: idiopathic atrophy, autoimmune, bilateral adrenal haemorrhage in sepsis (Waterhouse–Friderichsen syndrome), TB, pituitary insufficiency, metastatic deposits.

Excessive secretion

• Cushing's syndrome: *excess corticosteroid* due to steroid therapy, ACTH-producing pituitary tumour, adenoma or carcinoma of the adrenal cortex, ectopic ACTH production, e.g. oat cell carcinoma of lung.
• Conn's syndrome (primary hyperaldosteronism): *excess aldosterone* due to adenoma or carcinoma of adrenal cortex, bilateral cortical hyperplasia.
• Adrenogenital syndrome (adrenal virilism): caused by *excess androgen* production from adrenal cortical hyperplasia or a cortical tumour.
• Phaeochromocytoma: *excess catecholamines* due to adrenal medullary tumours, 95% are benign.

Clinical features

• Addison's disease: see opposite. Addisonian crisis: an acute collapse which may mimic an abdominal emergency.
• Cushing's syndrome: see opposite.
• Conn's syndrome, primary hyperaldosteronism: muscle weakness, paraesthesias, transient paralysis, tetany, polyuria, polydipsia, hypertension.
• Adrenogenital syndrome: virilization in female children, pseudohermaphroditism, precocious puberty, hirsuitism, baldness, acne.
• Phaeochromocytoma: see opposite.

Investigations

Basic principles

• Establish the 'endocrine' diagnosis by serum levels or suppressions/stimulation tests.
• Correct the endocrine abnormalities.
• Localize the cause by investigation and imaging.
• Consider if definitive (surgical) treatment is necessary.

Addison's disease

U+E ($\downarrow$ Na$^+$ <135 mmol/L, $\uparrow$ K$^+$ >5.0 mmol/L), fasting plasma glucose <2.78 mmol/L) and low plasma cortisol (<138 nmol/L). ACTH measurement and short Synacthen test to confirm diagnosis. Long Synacthen test to differentiate primary (adrenal) from secondary (pituitary) insufficiency.

Cushing's syndrome

• Elevated plasma cortisol (taken at 24.00 hours) and loss of diurnal variation.
• Low-dose dexamethasone suppression test to confirm diagnosis.
• High-dose test to distinguish adrenal from pituitary disease.
• Serum ACTH to identify secondary cause.

Conn's syndrome

U+E ($\downarrow$ K$^+$, normal or $\uparrow$ Na$^+$), raised serum aldosterone and normal renin levels.

Adrenogenital syndrome (adrenal virilism)

Elevated plasma DHEA, DHEA-sulphate, 17-hydroxyprogesterone, testosterone and androstenedione. Increase in 17-hydroxyprogesterone after Synacthen suggests adrenal hyperplasia. Failure of suppression of androgens production following dexamethasone suggests presence of androgen-secreting tumour.

Phaeochromocytoma

Plasma-free metanephrines is 99% sensitive. 24-hour urinary VMA and HVA may be used. (Consider MEN type II [parathyroid adenoma, medullary thyroid cancer, phaeochromocytoma]).

Localization imaging

• Helical CT and MRI: excellent for adrenal gland, retroperitoneum.
• ^{123}I-MIBG scan: neuroendocrine tumours (phaeochromocytoma).
• Arteriography and venous sampling: occasionally required.

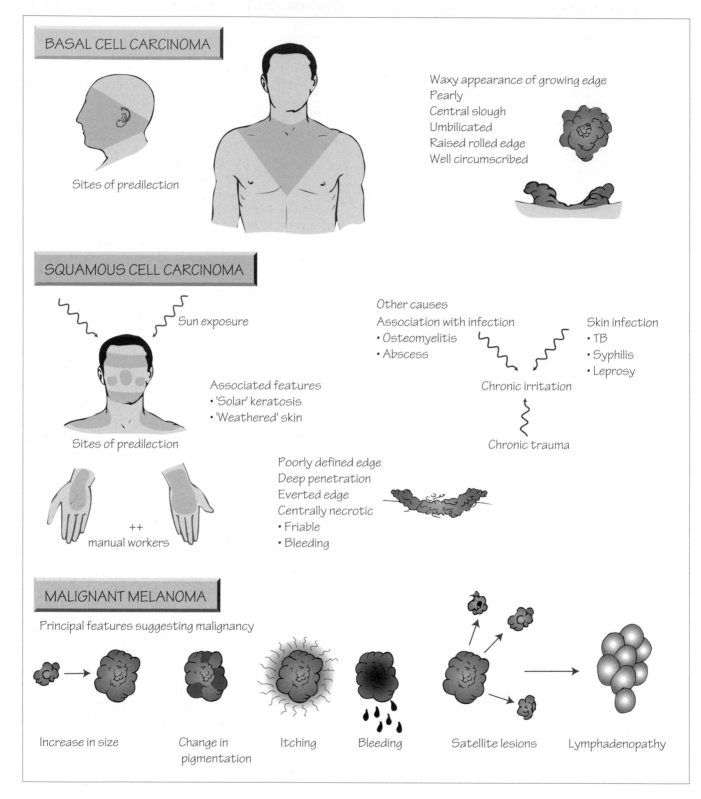

BASAL CELL CARCINOMA

Sites of predilection

Waxy appearance of growing edge
Pearly
Central slough
Umbilicated
Raised rolled edge
Well circumscribed

SQUAMOUS CELL CARCINOMA

Sun exposure

Associated features
• 'Solar' keratosis
• 'Weathered' skin

Sites of predilection

++
manual workers

Other causes
Association with infection
• Osteomyelitis
• Abscess

Chronic irritation

Chronic trauma

Skin infection
• TB
• Syphilis
• Leprosy

Poorly defined edge
Deep penetration
Everted edge
Centrally necrotic
• Friable
• Bleeding

MALIGNANT MELANOMA

Principal features suggesting malignancy

Increase in size   Change in pigmentation   Itching   Bleeding   Satellite lesions   Lymphadenopathy

Definition

Malignant lesions of epidermis of the skin—non-melanoma skin cancer (principally basal cell [BCC] and squamous cell [SCC] carcinomas) and malignant melanoma (MM).

Key points

- Protection from sun exposure reduces the risk of all forms of skin cancer dramatically ('*slip* on a shirt, *slop* on sunscreen, and *slap* on a hat').
- Not all MMs are pigmented.
- All 'moles' with suspicious features should be excision biopsied.
- The prognosis from early MM is excellent with surgery but late disease is usually fatal.

Epidemiology

Male : female 2 : 1 for BCC and SCC. Elderly males. Equal sex distribution and all adults for MM. Most common in fair skinned peoples (Irish, Scottish). All tumours common in areas of high annual sunshine (e.g. Australia, southern USA). BCC is the most common human cancer.

Aetiology

Predisposing factors:
- Exposure to sunlight—both UV-A (wave length 320–400 nm) and especially UV-B (290–320 nm) radiation damage skin. (UV-C [200–290 nm] does not penetrate the ozone layer.)
- Immunosuppression (high incidence after renal transplant).
- Radiation exposure (radiotherapy, among radiologists).
- Chemical carcinogens (hydrocarbons, arsenic, coal tar).
- Inherited disorders (albinism, xeroderma pigmentosum).
- Leukoplakia (clinical term to describe a white patch usually seen in the mouth).
- Chronic irritation: old burns, scars sites of radiotherapy, chronic ulcers (Marjolin's ulcer).
- Naevi (50% of MM arise in pre-existing benign pigmented lesions).
- Bowen's disease and erythroplasia of Queyrat.
- CDKN2A (*p16*) tumour suppressor gene mutation may be important in MM.

Pathology

Basal cell carcinoma
- Arises from basal cells of epidermis.
- Aggressive local spread—hence the name 'rodent ulcer'—but do not metastasize.

Squamous cell carcinoma
- Arises from keratinocytes in the epidermis.
- Spreads by local invasion, lymphatic spread and metastases. Large lesions (>2 cm) or deep lesions (>4 mm) may metastasize.

Malignant melanoma
- Arises from the melanocytes often in pre-existing naevi.

- Superficial spreading (70%), nodular types (10–15%) and lentigo maligna (10–15%).
- Radial and vertical growth phases. Lymphatic spread is to regional lymph nodes and haematogenous spread to liver, bone and brain.

Staging
- SCC: TNM (Stages I–IV)
- MM: Clarke's levels I–V and Breslow's tumour thickness (see below).

Clinical features

Basal cell carcinoma
Recurring, ulcerated, umbilicated skin lesion on forehead or face. Ulcer has a raised, pearl-coloured edge. Untreated, large areas of the face may be eroded (rodent ulcer).

Squamous cell carcinoma
Lesions (ulcers, fungating lesions with heaped-up edges) on exposed areas of the body.

Malignant melanoma
Pigmented lesions (occasionally not pigmented—amelanotic), 1 cm in diameter on lower limbs, feet, head and neck. Usually present as a change in a pigmented lesion: increasing size or pigmentation/bleeding/pain or itching/ulceration/satellite lesions.

Investigations
- Biopsy (usually excisional) of the lesion unless clinically certain (definitive surgery).
- For MM—helical CT scan for ?involved draining nodes, FNAC for palpable draining nodes, ?peroperative sentinel node biopsy using dye injection mapping.

Essential management

Basal cell carcinoma
- Curettage/cautery/cryotherapy/photodynamic therapy/topical chemotherapy (5-FU, imiquimod). These treatments may be suitable for small lesions.
- Surgical excision/radiotherapy—most effective treatments. Mohs' micrographic surgery (the tumour is removed layer by layer until completely gone as determined histologically) is the most effective treatment for high-risk facial BCC.

Squamous cell carcinoma
- Surgical excision/radiotherapy/cryosurgery for small lesions/Mohs' micrographic surgery.
- There is no topical treatment for SCC.

Malignant melanoma
- Excisional biopsy. If positive re-excision with margins depending on depth of tumour:
  - <1 mm thickness—1 cm margin
  - 1–4 mm thickness—2 cm margin
  - >4 mm thickness—at least 2 cm margin

• Lymph node dissection if **CT**, FNAC or sentinel node biopsy positive for metastases with no systemic disease.
• Adjuvant therapy may be indicated for patients with deep primary disease (>4 mm) or advanced disease. Immunotherapy (interferon-α2b), chemotherapy (dacarbazine) or combinations of these therapies.

2 Week wait referral criteria for suspected skin cancer

• Pigmented lesion + increased size/changed shape/changed colour/mixed colour/irregular/ulceration.
• Non-healing skin lesion.
• Biopsy-proven squamous carcinoma.
• New skin lesion in immunosuppressed.

Prognosis

• BCC, SCC prognosis is usually excellent—patients with SCC should be followed for 5 years.
• MM prognosis depends on staging:

Clarke's level	5-year survival (%)	Tumour thickness (mm)	5-year survival (%)
I (epidermis)	100	<0.76	98
II (papillary dermis)	90–100	0.76–1.49	95
III (papillary/reticular dermis)	80–90	1.50–2.49	80
IV (reticular dermis)	60–70	2.50–3.99	75
V (subcutaneous fat)	15–30	4.00–7.99	60
		>8.00	40

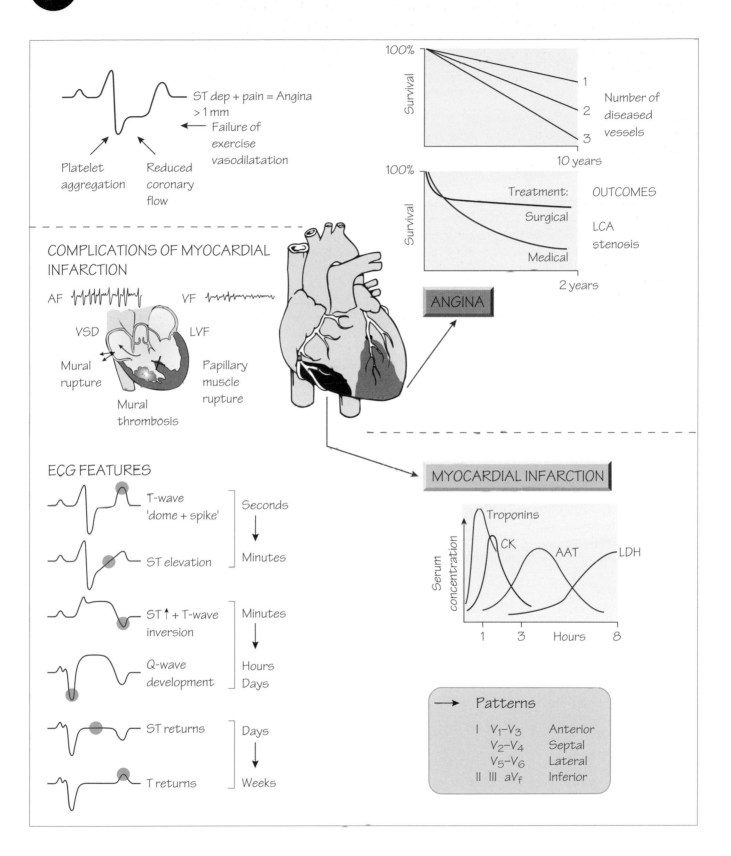

ST dep + pain = Angina
> 1 mm

Failure of exercise vasodilatation

Platelet aggregation

Reduced coronary flow

Survival 100%

1
2
3
Number of diseased vessels

10 years

Survival 100%

Treatment:
Surgical
Medical

OUTCOMES

LCA stenosis

2 years

ANGINA

COMPLICATIONS OF MYOCARDIAL INFARCTION

AF   VF

VSD   LVF

Mural rupture   Papillary muscle rupture

Mural thrombosis

MYOCARDIAL INFARCTION

Troponins
CK
AAT
LDH

Serum concentration

1   3   Hours   8

ECG FEATURES

T-wave 'dome + spike'   Seconds

ST elevation   Minutes

ST↑ + T-wave inversion   Minutes

Q-wave development   Hours / Days

ST returns   Days

T returns   Weeks

Patterns

I	V_1–V_3	Anterior
	V_2–V_4	Septal
	V_5–V_6	Lateral
II III aV$_f$		Inferior

Surgery at a Glance, 4e. By P. Grace and N.R. Borley. Published 2009 by Blackwell Publishing. ISBN 978-1-4051-8325-3.

Definition

Ischaemic heart disease is a common disorder caused by acute or chronic interruption of the blood supply to the myocardium, usually due to atherosclerosis of the coronary arteries, i.e. *coronary artery disease* (CAD). *Angina pectoris* (AP) is a pain in the centre of the chest induced by exercise and relieved by rest caused by coronary ischaemia. A *myocardial infarction* (MI) is death of a segment of heart muscle caused by ischaemia.

Key points

- Mortality from CAD is declining but CAD remains the principal cause of death in the Western world. One-third of patients with an acute MI will die.
- Urgent treatment with thrombolysis ('door-to-needle time' of <30 minutes) or intervention ('door-to-balloon time' of 120 minutes), antiplatelet agents, statins and cardioprotection reduces the risk of death from MI significantly.
- Serum troponins are highly sensitive and very specific for myocardial injury.
- Most atheromatous lesions that cause MI occlude <50% of the coronary artery lumen.
- Angina alone is rarely managed surgically (CABG).

Epidemiology

Male > female before 65 years. Increasing risk with increasing age up to 80 years. Most common cause of death in the Western world. Lower incidence of CAD in countries with Mediterranean diet (French paradox).

Aetiology

- Atherosclerosis and thrombosis.
- Thromboemboli (especially plaque rupture).
- Arteritis (e.g. periarteritis nodosa).
- Coronary artery spasm.
- Extension of aortic dissection/syphilitic aortitis.

Risk factors

- Family history.
- Hypertension.
- Diabetes mellitus.
- Metabolic syndrome.
- Hyperhomocysteinaemia.
- Cigarette smoking.
- Poor lipid profile (especially high LDL).
- Obesity.
- Type A personality.

Pathology

- The initiating event for the development of atherosclerosis may be vascular endothelial injury caused by altered haemodynamics, hyperglycaemia, dyslipidaemia, cigarette smoking, and ?infection (*Chlamydia pneumoniae*, *Helicobacter pylori*, *herpes simplex virus*).
- Reduction in coronary blood flow is critical when the lumen is decreased by 90%.

- Plaque rupture in non-critically stenosed arteries (<50% occlusion), precipitating local thrombosis and vessel occlusion, is frequently the cause of acute ischaemia.
- The heart muscle in the territory of the occluded vessel dies, i.e. MI. May be subendocardial or transmural.
- Angina pectoris results when the supply of O_2 to the heart muscle is unable to meet the increased demands, e.g. during exercise, cold, after a meal.

Clinical features

Spectrum of presentations: stable AP—unstable AP—acute MI—cardiac arrest—CCF—arrythmias.

Non-acute coronary artery disease

- Central chest pain on exertion, especially in cold weather, lasts 1–15 minutes.
- Radiates to neck, jaw, arms.
- Relieved by GTN.
- Usually no signs.

Acute coronary artery disease

- Severe central chest pain for >30 minutes' duration.
- Radiates to neck, jaw, arms.
- Not relieved by GTN.
- Signs of cardiogenic shock (sweating, dyspnoea, tachycardia, altered BP, ± CCF, murmurs).
- Arrhythmias.

Investigations

Non-acute coronary artery disease

- FBC and baseline chemistry.
- Lipid profile (total cholesterol, LDL, HDL, triglycerides).
- Inflammatory markers (CRP—in combination with LDL and HDL—identifies patients at risk of acute coronary syndromes).
- Thyroid function tests.
- Homocysteine levels.
- Chest X-ray: heart size.
- 12-lead ECG—ST segment changes.
- Exercise ECG and 24-hour ambulatory ECG monitoring.
- Myocardial perfusion nuclear (± stress) imaging—detects reversible myocardial perfusion defects.
- Coronary angiography, measurement of flow reserve and intravascular ultrasound assessment of atheromatous lesions.

Acute coronary syndromes (e.g. unstable angina, myocardial infarction)

- FBC, platelets, baseline chemistry (K^+ and Mg^{2+}) and creatinine, CRP.
- Serial ECG: Q waves, ST segment and T-wave changes.
- Serial serum markers: troponins (I and T), creatine kinase—myocardial band (CPK-MB), ischaemia-modified albumin, B-type natriuretic peptide.
- Chest X-ray: heart size, evidence of pulmonary oedema.
- Echocardiography (transthoracic for LV and valve function, transoesophageal for ?aortic dissection) ± stress echo (exercise or pharmacological).
- Angiography:

non-invasive—MRA, multidetector CT angiography
invasive—transluminal coronary angiography (cardiac catherization).

Complications of MI
- Arrhythmias.
- Cardiogenic shock.
- Myocardial rupture.
- Papillary muscle rupture causing mitral incompetence.
- Ventricular aneurysm.
- Pericarditis.
- Mural thrombosis and peripheral embolism.

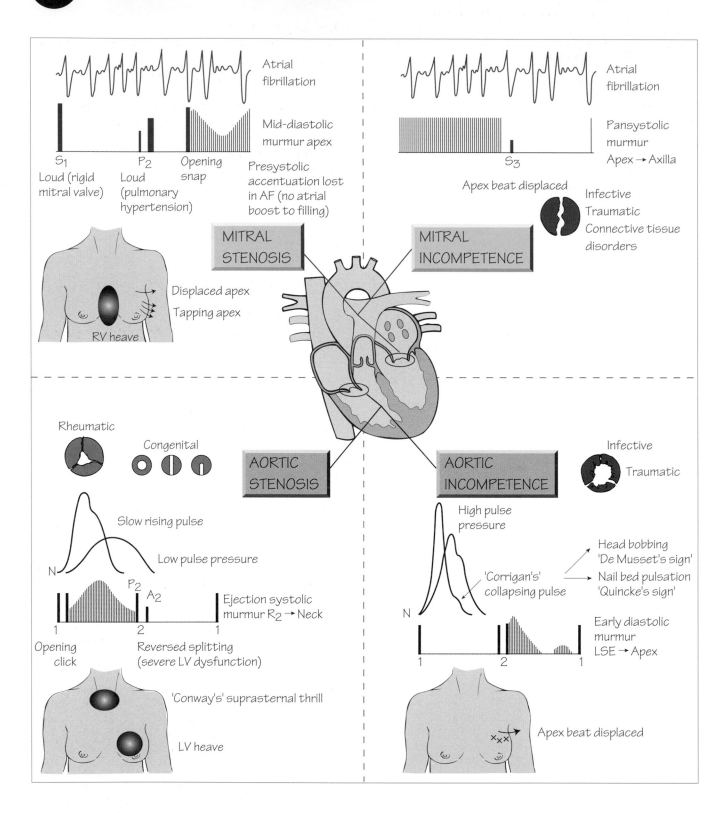

Atrial fibrillation

Mid-diastolic murmur apex

S_1 — Loud (rigid mitral valve)

P_2 — Loud (pulmonary hypertension)

Opening snap

Presystolic accentuation lost in AF (no atrial boost to filling)

MITRAL STENOSIS

Displaced apex
Tapping apex
RV heave

Atrial fibrillation

Pansystolic murmur
Apex → Axilla

S_3

Apex beat displaced

MITRAL INCOMPETENCE

Infective
Traumatic
Connective tissue disorders

Rheumatic

Congenital

AORTIC STENOSIS

Slow rising pulse

Low pulse pressure

P_2 A_2

Ejection systolic murmur R_2 → Neck

Opening click

Reversed splitting (severe LV dysfunction)

'Conway's' suprasternal thrill

LV heave

AORTIC INCOMPETENCE

Infective
Traumatic

High pulse pressure

'Corrigan's' collapsing pulse

Head bobbing 'De Musset's sign'

Nail bed pulsation 'Quincke's sign'

Early diastolic murmur LSE → Apex

Apex beat displaced

Definition

Valvular heart disease is defined as a group of congenital or acquired conditions characterized by damage to one or more of the heart valves, resulting in deranged blood flow through the heart chambers.

Epidemiology

Rheumatic fever is still a major problem in developing countries, while congenital heart disease occurs in 8–10 cases per 1000 live births worldwide.

Aetiology

• Congenital valve abnormalities.
• Rheumatic fever.
• Infective endocarditis.
• Degenerative valve disease.

Pathology

• Rheumatic fever—*immune-mediated acute inflammation* affecting the heart valves due to a cross-reaction between antigens of group A α-haemolytic *Streptococcus* and cardiac proteins.
• Disease may make the valve orifice smaller (*stenosis*) or unable to close properly (*incompetence* or *regurgitation*) or both.
• Stenosis causes a *pressure load* while regurgitation causes a *volume load* on the heart chamber immediately proximal to it with upstream and downstream effects.

Clinical features

Aortic stenosis

(Senile degeneration most common cause.)
• Angina pectoris.
• Dizziness, syncope.
• Left heart failure.
• Slow upstroke arterial pulse.
• Precordial systolic thrill (second right ICS).
• Harsh midsystolic ejection murmur (second right ICS).

Aortic regurgitation

(Congenital, rheumatic, infective endocarditis most common causes.)
• Dyspnoea, palpitations.
• Congestive cardiac failure.
• Wide pulse pressure.
• Water-hammer pulse.
• Decrescendo diastolic murmur (lower LSE).

Mitral stenosis

(Rheumatic and congenital most common causes.)
• Pulmonary hypertension.
• Paroxysmal nocturnal dyspnoea.
• Atrial fibrillation.
• Malar flush
• Loud first heart sound and opening snap.

• Low-pitched diastolic murmur with presystolic accentuation at the apex.

Mitral regurgitation

(Functional, degenerative, rheumatic, infective carditis most common causes.)
• Dyspnoea, chronic fatigue, palpitations.
• Pulmonary oedema.
• Apex laterally displaced, hyperdynamic praecordium.
• Apical pansystolic murmur radiating to axilla.

Tricuspid stenosis

(Rheumatic most common cause—usually aortic or mitral disease as well.)
• Fatigue.
• Peripheral oedema.
• Liver enlargement/ascites.
• Prominent JVP with large a waves.
• Lung fields are clear.
• Rumbling diastolic murmur (lower left sternal border).

Tricuspid regurgitation

(Functional, rheumatic, infective carditis most common causes.)
• Chronic fatigue.
• Hepatomegaly/ascites.
• Peripheral oedema.
• Right ventricular heave.
• Prominent JVP with large v waves.
• Pansystolic murmur (subxiphoid area).

Investigations

• ECG.
• Chest X-ray.
• Echocardiography and colour Doppler techniques.
• Cardiac catheterization with measurement of transvalvular gradients.

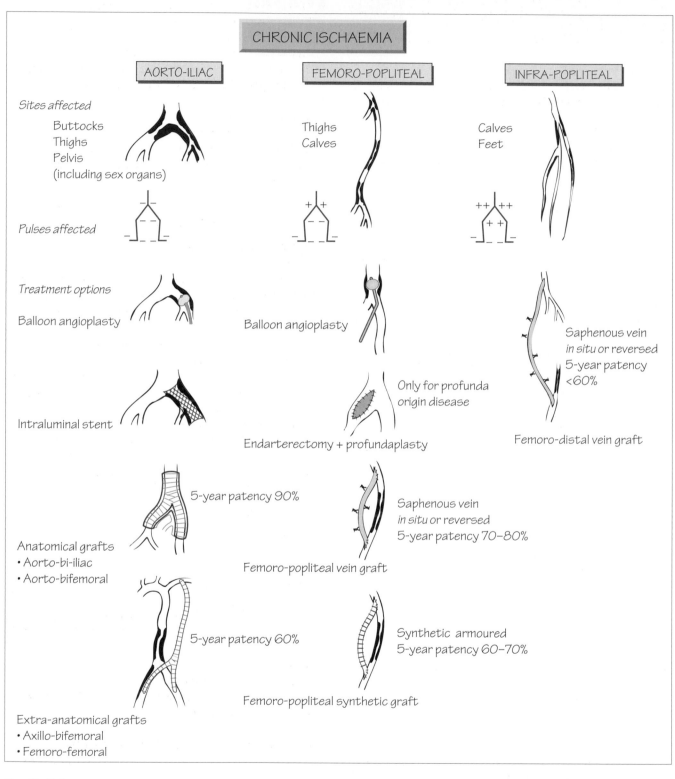

Definition

Peripheral arterial disease (PAD) (*peripheral arterial occlusive disease, peripheral occlusive vascular disease*) is a common disorder caused by acute or chronic interruption of blood supply to the limbs, usually due to atherosclerosis.

Key points

• All patients with PAD require screening for associated coronary or carotid disease.

Epidemiology

Male > female before 65 years. Increased risk with increased age. Affects 10% of population >65 years in Western world.

Aetiology

• Atherosclerosis and thrombosis.
• Embolism (80% cardiac in origin, microemboli cause 'blue toe syndrome').
• Vascular trauma.
• Vasculitis (e.g. Buerger's disease).

Risk factors

Cigarette smoking, hypertension, hyperlipidaemia, diabetes mellitus, family history.

Pathology

Reduction in blood flow to the peripheral tissues results in ischaemia which may be acute or chronic. Critical Ischaemia Is present when tissue viability cannot be sustained (i.e., tissue loss, rest pain for 2 weeks, ankle pressure 50 mmHg).

Clinical features
Fontaine classification

• Stage I, asymptomatic.
• Stage II, intermitent claudication.
• Stage III, rest pain/nocturnal pain.
• Stage IV, necrosis/gangrene.

Chronic ischaemia (see Chapter 19)

• Intermittent claudication in calf (femoral disease), thigh (iliac disease) or buttock (aorto-iliac disease).
• Cold peripheries and prolonged capillary refill time.
• Rest pain, especially at night.
• Venous guttering.
• Absent pulses.
• Arterial ulcers, especially over pressure points (heels, toes).
• Knee contractures.
  Leriche's syndrome (intermittent claudication, impotence, absent femoral pulses) indicates aortic occlusion.

Acute ischaemia (see Chapter 21)

• Pain.
• Pallor.
• Pulselessness.
• Paraesthesia and paralysis—indicate limb-threatening ischaemia that requires immediate treatment.
• 'Perishing' cold.
• 'Pistol shot' onset.
• Mottling.
• Muscle rigidity.

Investigations
Chronic ischaemia

• ABI (normal >0.9) at rest and postexercise on treadmill.
• Digital pressures (normal toe pressure >50 mmHg)
• FBC (exclude polycythaemia).
• Doppler waveform analysis.
• Digital plethysmography (in diabetes).
• Duplex ultrasound e.g. assessing a stenosis in the femoral artery.
• Angiography (MRA, CTA or catherter angiography).

Acute ischaemia

• ECG, cardiac enzymes.
• Angiography (?), may be performed peroperatively.
• Find source of embolism. Holter monitoring. Echocardiograph. Ultrasound aorta for AAA.

Prognosis
Non-disabling claudication

>65% respond to conservative management. The rest require more aggressive treatment.

Disabling claudication/critical ischaemia

• Angioplasty (may be subintimal) and bypass surgery overall give good results.
• The more distal the disease the poorer the results of intervention.

Acute ischaemia

• Limb salvage 85%; mortality 10–15%.

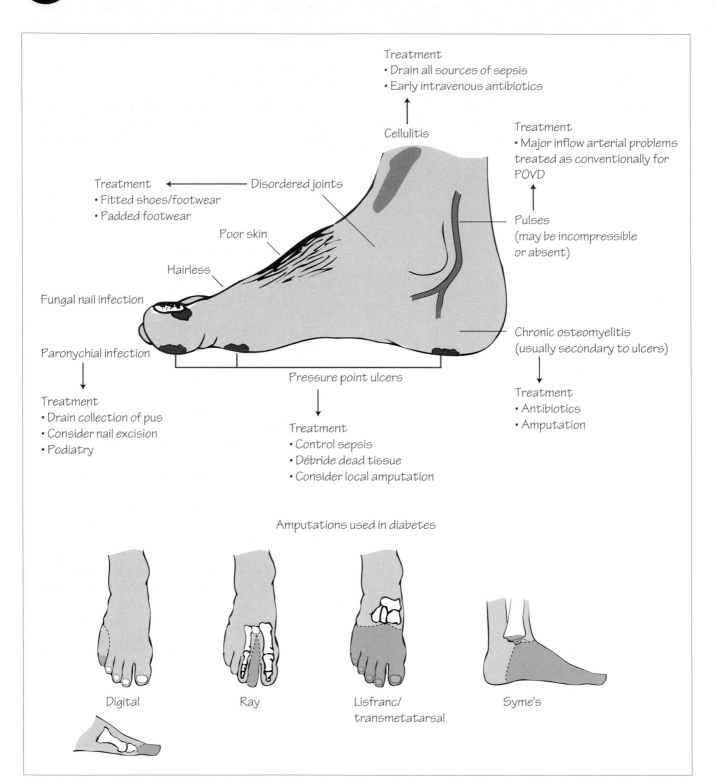

Treatment
• Drain all sources of sepsis
• Early intravenous antibiotics

Cellulitis

Treatment
• Major inflow arterial problems treated as conventionally for POVD

Disordered joints

Treatment
• Fitted shoes/footwear
• Padded footwear

Poor skin

Hairless

Pulses
(may be incompressible or absent)

Fungal nail infection

Paronychial infection

Chronic osteomyelitis
(usually secondary to ulcers)

Pressure point ulcers

Treatment
• Drain collection of pus
• Consider nail excision
• Podiatry

Treatment
• Control sepsis
• Débride dead tissue
• Consider local amputation

Treatment
• Antibiotics
• Amputation

Amputations used in diabetes

Digital

Ray

Lisfranc/
transmetatarsal

Syme's

Definition

The term *diabetic foot* refers to a spectrum of foot disorders ranging from ulceration to gangrene occurring in people with diabetes mellitus (DM) as a result of peripheral neuropathy or ischaemia, or both.

Key points

- Prevention is all important with diabetic feet.
- All infections should be treated aggressively to reduce the risk of tissue loss.
- Treat major vessel POVD as normal—improve 'inflow' to the foot.
- Limb loss is a significant risk in patients with diabetic foot ulcers.

Pathophysiology

Three distinct processes lead to the problem of the diabetic foot:
- *Ischaemia*: macro- and microangiopathy. Higher incidence of atherosclerosis with DM.
- *Neuropathy*: sensory, motor and autonomic—multifactorial in origin.
- *Sepsis*: the glucose-saturated tissue promotes bacterial growth.

Clinical features

Neuropathic features

- Sensory disturbances—loss of vibratory and position sense.
- Trophic skin changes.
- Plantar ulceration.
- Degenerative osteoarthropathy (Charcot's joints)—occurs in 2% of DM patients.
- Pulses often present.
- Sepsis (bacterial/fungal).

Ischaemic features

- Rest pain.
- Painful ulcers over pressure areas.
- History of intermittent claudication.
- Absent pulses.
- Sepsis (bacterial/fungal).

Investigations

- FBC: leucocytosis.
- Serum glucose and gylcosylated Hb (HbA1c): diabetic control may be poor due to sepsis.
- Non-invasive vascular tests: ABI, segmental pressure, digital pressure. ABI may be falsely elevated due to medial sclerosis. Digital pressures more accurate in patients with DM.
- X-ray of foot or CT/MRI may show osteomyelitis or abscess.
- Arteriography (MRA, CTA or catheter angiography).

Essential management

Should be undertaken jointly by surgeon and physician as diabetic foot may precipitate diabetic ketoacidosis. Diabetic patients should be prescribed an antiplatelet agent and a statin.

Prevention

Do
- Carefully wash and dry feet daily.
- Inspect feet daily.
- Take meticulous care of toenails.
- Use antifungal powder.

Do not
- Walk barefoot.
- Wear ill-fitting shoes.
- Use a hot water bottle.
- Ignore any foot injury.

Neuropathic disease

- Control infection with antibiotics effective against both aerobes and anaerobes.
- Wide local excision and drainage of necrotic tissue ± skin grafting later.
- Pressure offloading: avoid weight-bearing on the wound/ulcer—special footwear, total contact casting.
- These measures usually result in healing.

Ischaemic disease

- Formal assessment of the vascular tree by angiography and reconstitution of the blood supply to the foot (either by angioplasty or bypass surgery) must be achieved before the local measures will work.
- After restoration of blood supply treat as for neuropathic disease.

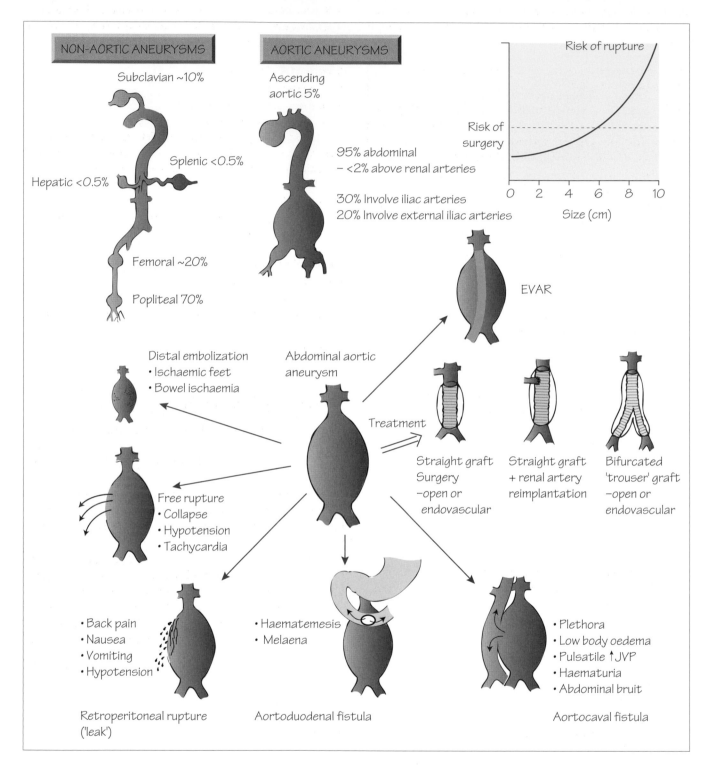

Definitions

An *aneurysm* is a permanent localized dilatation of an artery to the extent that the affected artery is 1.5 times its normal diameter. A *pseudo* or *false aneurysm* is an expanding pulsating haematoma in continuity with a vessel lumen. It does not have an epithelial lining.

Key points

- Screening for AAA by ultrasound in men aged 65–79 years results in a significant reduction in mortality from AAA. No benefit from screening in women or younger men.
- All patients with other vascular disease should be examined for AAA.
- There is no medical treatment for AAA.
- Regular monitoring of size helps determine timing for elective intervention.
- Mortality for elective surgery is reduced by careful patient evaluation for hidden coronary or pulmonary disease.

Sites

Abdominal aorta, iliac, femoral and popliteal arteries. Cerebral and thoracic aneurysms are less common.

Aetiology

- Atherosclerosis.
- Familial (abnormal collagenase or elastase activity).
- Congenital (cerebral [berry] aneurysm).
- Bacterial aortitis (mycotic aneurysm).
- Syphilitic aortitis (thoracic aneurysm).

Risk factors

- Cigarette smoking.
- Hypertension.
- Hyperlipidaemia.

Pathology

- Aneurysms increase in size in line with the law of Laplace ($T = RP$), T = tension on the arterial wall, R = radius of artery, P = blood pressure. Increasing tension leads to rupture.
- Thrombus from within an aneurysm may be a source of peripheral emboli.
- Popliteal aneurysms may undergo complete thrombosis leading to acute leg ischaemia.
- Aneurysms may be fusiform (AAA, popliteal) or saccular (thoracic, cerebral).

Clinical features of AAA

Asymptomatic

The vast majority have no symptoms and are found incidentally. This has led to the description of an AAA as 'a U-boat in the belly' and the development of screening programmes.

Symptomatic

- Back pain from pressure on the vertebral column.
- Rapid expansion causes flank or back pain.
- Rupture causes collapse, back pain and an ill-defined mass.
- Erosion into IVC causes CCF, loud abdominal bruit (machinery murmur), lower limb ischaemia and gross oedema.

Investigations

Detection of AAA

- Physical examination: not accurate.
- Plain abdominal X-ray: aortic calcification.
- Ultrasonography: best way of detecting and measuring aneurysm size—many localities have effective U/S-based screening services to reduce acute presentations of rupture.
- CT scan: provides good information regarding relationship between AAA and renal arteries.
- Angiography: needed for anatomical detail for planning endovascular repair.

Determination of fitness for surgery

- History and examination.
- ECG ± stress testing.
- Radionuclide cardiac scanning (MUGA or stress thallium scan).
- Pulmonary function tests.
- U+E and creatinine for renal assessment.

Essential management

- Endovascular or surgical repair is the treatment of choice for AAA.
- AAA of ≥5.5 cm should be repaired electively as they have a high rate of rupture. AAA <5.5 cm may be monitored with serial ultrasound or CT examinations every 6 months.
- Endovascular repair with graft/stent devices is a commonly used method of repair In many patients now. 30-day mortality 2%.
- Surgical repair with inlay of a synthetic graft (laparoscopic or open) may be used for suitable patients, especially those not suitable for endovascular repair. 30-day mortality 5%.
- Ruptured AAA require immediate surgical (or endovascular) repair (perioperative mortality 50%, but 70% of patients die before they get to hospital so that overall mortality is 85%).

Prognosis

Most patients do well after surviving AAA repair and have an excellent quality of life.

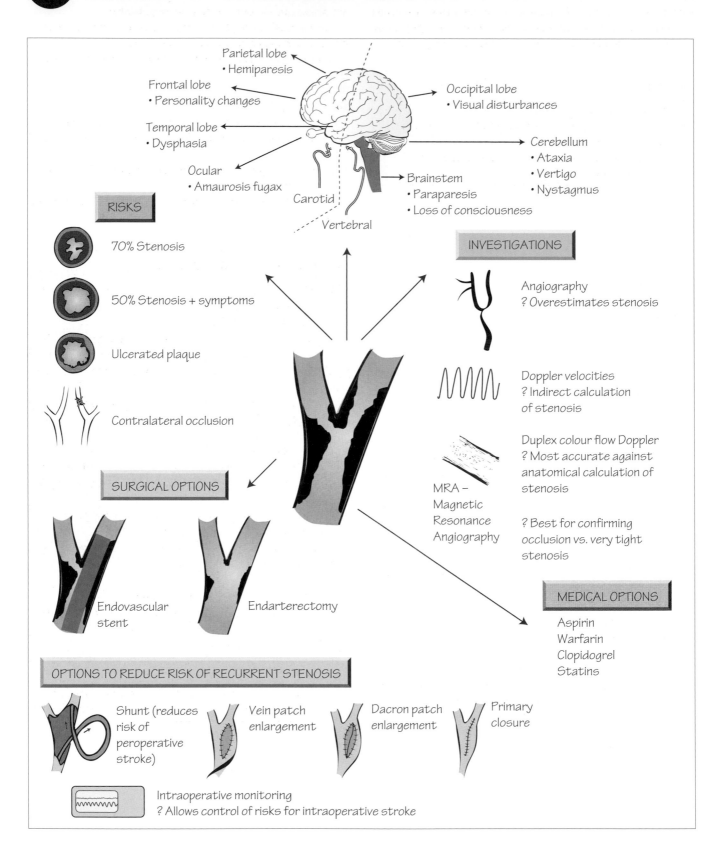

RISKS

70% Stenosis

50% Stenosis + symptoms

Ulcerated plaque

Contralateral occlusion

Parietal lobe
• Hemiparesis

Frontal lobe
• Personality changes

Temporal lobe
• Dysphasia

Ocular
• Amaurosis fugax

Carotid

Vertebral

Occipital lobe
• Visual disturbances

Cerebellum
• Ataxia
• Vertigo
• Nystagmus

Brainstem
• Paraparesis
• Loss of consciousness

INVESTIGATIONS

Angiography
? Overestimates stenosis

Doppler velocities
? Indirect calculation
of stenosis

Duplex colour flow Doppler
? Most accurate against
anatomical calculation of
stenosis

MRA –
Magnetic
Resonance
Angiography

? Best for confirming
occlusion vs. very tight
stenosis

SURGICAL OPTIONS

Endovascular
stent

Endarterectomy

MEDICAL OPTIONS

Aspirin
Warfarin
Clopidogrel
Statins

OPTIONS TO REDUCE RISK OF RECURRENT STENOSIS

Shunt (reduces
risk of
peroperative
stroke)

Vein patch
enlargement

Dacron patch
enlargement

Primary
closure

Intraoperative monitoring
? Allows control of risks for intraoperative stroke

Definition

Extracranial arterial disease is a common disorder characterized by atherosclerosis of the carotid or vertebral arteries resulting in cerebral (*stroke, TIA*), ocular (*amaurosis fugax*) or cerebellar (*vertigo, ataxia, drop attacks*) ischaemic symptoms.

Key points

- All patients with transient neurological symptoms should undergo ultrasound examination for carotid disease—clinical examination is not accurate.
- Targeted carotid endarterectomy offers optimal risk benefit in stroke prevention.

Epidemiology

Male > female before 65 years. Increasing risk with increasing age.

Aetiology

- Atherosclerosis and thrombosis.
- Thromboemboli.
- Fibromuscular dysplasia.

Risk factors

- Cigarette smoking.
- Hypertension.
- Hyperlipidaemia.

Pathophysiology

- The most common extracranial lesion is an atherosclerotic plaque at the carotid bifurcation. Platelet aggregation and subsequent *platelet embolization* cause ocular or cerebral symptoms.
- Symptoms due to *flow reduction* are rare in the carotid territory, but vertebrobasilar symptoms are usually flow-related. Reversed flow in the vertebral artery in the presence of ipsilateral subclavian occlusion leads to cerebral symptoms as the arm 'steals' blood from the cerebellum—subclavian steal syndrome.

Clinical features

- Cerebral symptoms (contralateral):
  motor (weakness, clumsiness or paralysis of a limb)
  sensory (numbness, paraesthesia)
  speech-related (receptive or expressive dysphasia).
- Ocular symptoms (ipsilateral): amaurosis fugax (transient loss of vision described as 'a veil coming down over the visual field').

- Cerebral (or ocular) symptoms may be transitory (a *transient ischaemic attack* is a focal neurological or ocular deficit lasting not more than 24 hours) or permanent (a *stroke*).
- Vertebrobasilar symptoms: vertigo, ataxia, dizziness, syncope, bilateral paraesthesia, visual hallucinations.
- A *bruit* may be heard over a carotid artery, but it is an unreliable indicator of pathology.

Investigations

- Duplex scanning: B-mode scan and Doppler ultrasonic velocitometry: method of choice for assessing degree of carotid stenosis.
- Carotid angiography: now often performed as MRA, which is safer than standard angiography.
- CT or MRI brain scan: demonstrate the presence of a cerebral infarct.

Essential management

Medical

- Smoking cessation.
- Blood pressure control.
- Antiplatelet agent: inhibits platelet aggregation for the life of the platelet (75 mg/day aspirin or 75 mg/day clopidogrel).
- All patients with evidence of vascular disease should be prescribed a statin.
- Anticoagulation is indicated in patients with cardiac embolic disease.

Interventional

- Carotid endarterectomy (CEA) (+ maximum medical therapy). Most benefit is achieved if carotid endarterectomy is performed within 2 weeks on onset of symptoms.
- Carotid angioplasty and stent (CAS) using a protection device to prevent distal embolization (+ maximum medical therapy). Role is controversial. Useful in 'hostile neck', e.g. previous surgery or radiotherapy.

Indications for carotid endarterectomy

- Carotid distribution TIA or stroke with good recovery after 1-month delay:
  >70% ipsilateral stenosis
  >50% ipsilateral stenosis with ulceration.
- Asymptomatic carotid stenosis >80% (controversial).
- Carotid intervention (CEA or CAS) has about 3–5% morbidity and mortality.

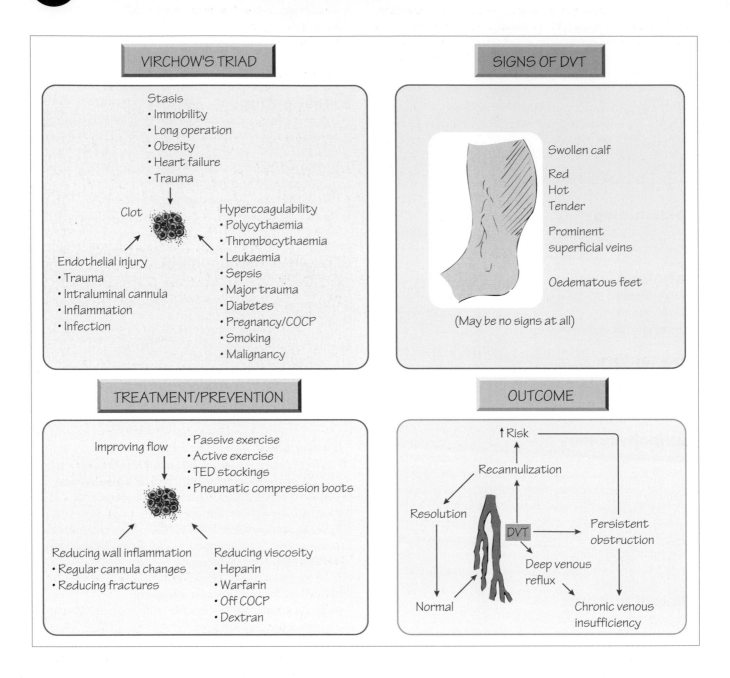

VIRCHOW'S TRIAD

Stasis
• Immobility
• Long operation
• Obesity
• Heart failure
• Trauma

Clot

Hypercoagulability
• Polycythaemia
• Thrombocythaemia
• Leukaemia
• Sepsis
• Major trauma
• Diabetes
• Pregnancy/COCP
• Smoking
• Malignancy

Endothelial injury
• Trauma
• Intraluminal cannula
• Inflammation
• Infection

SIGNS OF DVT

Swollen calf

Red
Hot
Tender

Prominent
superficial veins

Oedematous feet

(May be no signs at all)

TREATMENT/PREVENTION

Improving flow
• Passive exercise
• Active exercise
• TED stockings
• Pneumatic compression boots

Reducing wall inflammation
• Regular cannula changes
• Reducing fractures

Reducing viscosity
• Heparin
• Warfarin
• Off COCP
• Dextran

OUTCOME

↑Risk

Recannulization

Resolution

DVT

Persistent
obstruction

Deep venous
reflux

Normal

Chronic venous
insufficiency

Definitions

A *deep venous thrombosis* (DVT) is a condition in which the blood in the deep veins of the legs or pelvis clots. It can also occasionally occur in the upper limbs. Embolization of the thrombus results in a *pulmonary embolus* (PE) while local venous damage may lead to chronic venous insufficiency (CVI) also known as post-thrombotic or postphlebitic syndrome or limb.

> ### Key points
>
> - All patients in hospital should be considered for mechanical and pharmacological DVT prophylaxis.
> - Have a low threshold of investigation for DVT in bed-bound patients.
> - In clinically suspected DVT or PE, heparin should be commenced (unless strongly indicated) until diagnosis is excluded by diagnostic imaging.
> - Recurrent DVT may lead to chronic disabling post-phlebitic limb.
> - DVT may be the first manifestation of an occult malignancy.

Epidemiology

DVT is extremely common among medical and surgical patients, affecting 10–30% of all general surgical patients over 40 years who undergo a major operation. PE is a common cause of sudden death in hospital patients (0.5–3.0% of patients die from PE).

Aetiology

Virchow's triad (see opposite)

Pathology

- Aggregation of platelets in venous valve cusps (area of maximum stasis or injury).
- Activation of clotting cascade producing fibrin.
- Fibrin production overwhelms the natural anticoagulant/fibrinolytic system.
- Natural history: complete resolution vs. PE vs. CVI.

Clinical features

Deep venous thrombosis

- Asymptomatic.
- Calf tenderness or aching, ankle oedema, mild pyrexia.
- Phlegmasia alba/caerulea dolens.

Pulmonary embolism

- Dyspnoea ± pleuritic chest pain.
- Tachycardia and tachypnoea.
- Cough ± haemoptysis, fever.
- Massive PE causes circulatory arrest.

Chronic venous insufficiency (see Chapter 70)

- History of DVT.

- Aching limb.
- Leg swelling and varicose veins.
- Venous eczema and lipodermatosclerosis.
- Venous ulceration.
- Inverted bottle-shaped leg.

Diagnosis and investigations

Wells' clinical prediction score for DVT (quantifies probability of DVT).	
Active cancer	+1
Post bed rest for >3 days or major surgery	+1
Entire leg swelling	+1
Pitting oedema	+1
Collateral superficial veins (not venous valves)	+1
Paralysis or recent POP lower limb	+1
Tender over deep venous system	+1
Calf swelling >3 cm over other leg	+1
Previous documented DVT	+1
Alternative diagnosis more likely	−2
Probability of DVT: high ≥3, medium 1 or 2, low ≥0.	

Deep venous thrombosis

- D-dimers (byproduct of fibrinolysis—95% sensitivity. A negative test excludes DVT in low to moderate risk patients (Wells' score <2) but a positive test does not confirm a DVT. A duplex image is required if D-dimers positive).
- Duplex imaging—gold standard for DVT diagnosis now. Excellent for femoral and popliteal DVT, less accurate for calf and iliac—MRI is more accurate in these but expensive.
- Impedence phlethysmography is used occasionally. Good for diagnosis of proximal vein thrombosis. (Detects reduced venous outflow from and increased volume of affected limb.)
- CT venography may used if ilio-femoral DVT is suspected.

Pulmonary embolism

- ECG: tachycardia, S1, Q3, T3 or right bundle branch block, atrial fibrillation.
- WBC may be elevated.
- D-dimer testing.
- Pulse oximetry, arterial blood gases: hypoxia, hypocapnia.
- Chest X-ray: atelectasis, small pleural effusion, elevated hemi-diaphragm, infiltrates.
- Nuclear scintigraphic V/Q scanning of the lung.
- Multidetector CTA—if available, is the preferred primary diagnostic modality for PE.

Chronic venous insufficiency

- Colour duplex imaging.
- Plethysmography.
- Ascending ± descending venography.
- Ambulatory venous pressure.

Essential management

Prophylaxis against DVT

Indications

Presence of risk factors (see above).

Methods

• Mechanical compression: (TED) stockings or intermittent pneumatic compression devices.

• Pharmacological:

low dose unfractionated heparin (LDUH)—5000 IU s.c., b.i.d.

low molecular weight heparin (LMWH)—dose depends on drug—better prevention but more more expensive than LDUH

fondaparinux (Factor Xa inhibitor)—2.5 mg/day

warfarin and newer anticoagulants (hirudin, lepirudin).

Definitive treatment

Deep venous thrombosis

• Anticoagulation for 12 weeks:

initial Rx: IV unfractionated heparin (check efficacy with APTT) *or* s.c. LMWH (no APTT monitoring required)

maintenance: oral anticoagulation (warfarin) in non-pregnant patients (target INR 2.0–3.0). In pregnant use LMWH

• Compression stockings: graduated-compression below-knee elastic stockings × 2 years reduces risk of developing postphlebitic limb.

(• Thrombolysis: may be useful in selected patients with ilio-femoral DVT—haemorrhage a major side-effect. Thrombectomy rarely performed.)

Pulmonary embolism

Emergency treatment:

• Fibrinolysis should be considered in all patients unless specifically contraindications. Definite indications: haemodynamically unstable, right heart strain, likely recurrent PE.

• Prompt anticoagulation with heparin.

• Oxygen therapy.

• Pulmonary embolectomy or extracorporeal membrane oxygenation may be indicated.

Later management:

• Anticoagulation for at least 6 months.

• Look for source of embolus.

• Compression stockings.

• IVC filters for recurrent PE despite treatment, anticoagulation treatment contraindicated, 'high risk' DVTs.

Chronic venous insufficiency

• Limb elevation.

• Compression: four-layer bandaging to achieve ulcer healing. Graduated compression stockings to maintain limb.

• Varicose veins should be treated if there is an unobstructed deep venous system.

• Venous valvuoplasty or venous transposition has been used for deep venous incompetence.

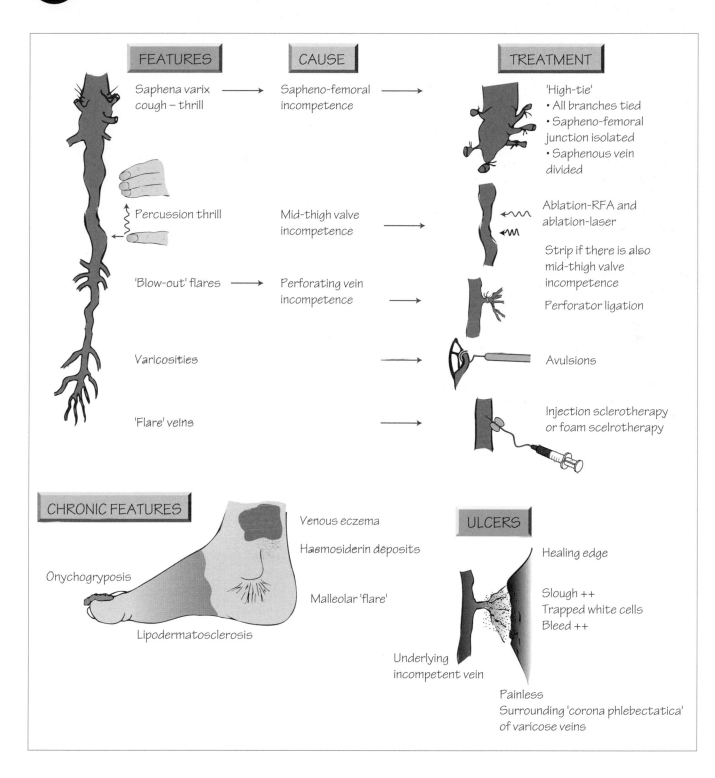

FEATURES

Saphena varix
cough – thrill

Percussion thrill

'Blow-out' flares

Varicosities

'Flare' veins

CAUSE

Sapheno-femoral
incompetence

Mid-thigh valve
incompetence

Perforating vein
incompetence

TREATMENT

'High-tie'
• All branches tied
• Sapheno-femoral
  junction isolated
• Saphenous vein
  divided

Ablation-RFA and
ablation-laser

Strip if there is also
mid-thigh valve
incompetence

Perforator ligation

Avulsions

Injection sclerotherapy
or foam scelrotherapy

CHRONIC FEATURES

Onychogryposis

Lipodermatosclerosis

Venous eczema

Haemosiderin deposits

Malleolar 'flare'

ULCERS

Healing edge

Slough ++
Trapped white cells
Bleed ++

Underlying
incompetent vein

Painless
Surrounding 'corona phlebectatica'
of varicose veins

Surgery at a Glance, 4e. By P. Grace and N.R. Borley. Published 2009 by Blackwell Publishing. ISBN 978-1-4051-8325-3. **163**

Definition

Varicose veins are tortuous, dilated, prominent, superficial veins in the lower limbs, often in the anatomical distribution of the long and short saphenous veins.

> ### Key points
>
> • Modern treatments for varicose veins include surgery (sapheno-femoral disconnection, stripping and multiple avulsions), radiofrequency or laser ablation and foam sclerotherapy.
> • Beware non-anatomical or atypical varicose veins in the young adult (congenital causes).
> • Colour duplex imaging (B-mode greyscale image + Doppler waveform) is the standard method of assessing venous anatomy and function.
> • Pre-treatment duplex imaging should be considered in all patients undergoing treatment for varicose veins.

Epidemiology

Very common in the Western world, affecting about 50% of the adult population.

Aetiology

• Primary or familial varicose veins.
• Pregnancy (progesterone causes passive dilatation of veins).
• Secondary to postphlebitic limb (perforator failure).
• Congenital:
  Klippel–Trenaunay syndrome (port-wine stain, varicose veins, bony and soft tissue hypertrophy involving an extremity)
  Parkes–Weber syndrome (cutaneous flush with underlying multiple microarteriovenous fistulas, in association with soft tissue and skeletal hypertrophy of the affected limb)
• Iatrogenic: following formation of an arteriovenous fistula.

Pathophysiology

Venous valve failure, usually at the sapheno-femoral or sapheno-popliteal junction (and sometimes in perforating veins), results in increased venous pressure in the LSV or SSV with progressive vein dilatation and further valve disruption.

Clinical features

CEAP classification for lower extremity venous disease

• Clinical
  - 0 No visible or palpable signs of venous disease
  - 1 Telangiectasia, reticular veins
  - 2 Varicose veins
  - 3 Oedema without skin changes
  - 4 Skin changes: (a) pigmentation, venous eczema; (b) lipodermatosclerosis
  - 5 Healed ulcer venous ulcer
  - 6 Active venous ulcer
  - s Symptomatic (ache, pain, tightness, irritation, heaviness, cramp)
  - a Asymptomatic

• **Etiology:** Ec (congenital), Ep (primary), Es (secondary—post-thrombotic), En (no cause).
• **Anatomy:** As (superficial), Ap (perforator), Ad (deep), An (no venous location identified).
• **Pathophysiological:** Pr (reflux), Po (obstruction), Pr,o reflux + obstruction, Pn (no venous pathophysiology.

The date of CEAP assessment should also be recorded, e.g. C4a,s, Ep, As Pr (28-7-2008).

Investigations

The level of investigations depends on the severity of the disease:

• Level I: history and clinical examination (Trendelenburg tests) + hand-help Doppler.
• Level II: non-invasive vascular—colour duplex scanning ± phlethysmography.
• Level III: more complex imaging (CT or MRI), ascending or decending venograph, invasive venous pressure measurements.

Essential management

General
- Avoid long periods of standing or sitting.
- Weight loss and exercise.
- Elevate limbs and use skin lotions.
- Compression: wear support hosiery.

Specific

Surgical ablation (standard method of treatment until recently)
- With the patient standing, the dilated veins are carefully marked with an indelible marker.
- The LSV or SSV is surgically disconnected from the superficial femoral or popliteal vein, respectively.
- The elongated veins are removed via multiple stab incisions and long segments above the knee are removed using a 'vein stripper'.
- Compression stockings are worn for several weeks and exercise is encouraged.
- Standard surgery improves quality of life and is cost-effective.

Endovenous ablation
- Endovenous ablation involves placement of an energy-delivering catheter (radiofrequency or laser) into the vein to be treated (LSV or SSV) after infiltration of anaesthesia along the course of the vein. Ablation is achieved by heat produced by the energy source.
- Achieve occlusion rates of 80–90%. Can be performed under LA and is safe. Expensive.

Ultrasound guided foam sclerotherapy
- A foam is prepared by mixing the sclerosing agent (polidocanol and ethanol) with air. The sclerosant is injected into the vein (under ultrasound guidance for larger veins) causing chemical thrombophlebitis and occlusion. The vein must be compressed to press the walls together and prevent recanalization.
- Occlusion rates of 80%. Outpatient procedure. Minimally invasive. Cheap. Very useful for small veins but has been used to obliterate LSV and SSV. Treatments can be repeated. Extravasation of agent can cause pigmentation or skin necrosis. Rarely foam may enter the arterial circulation via a patent foramen ovale and cause visual or cerebral symptoms.

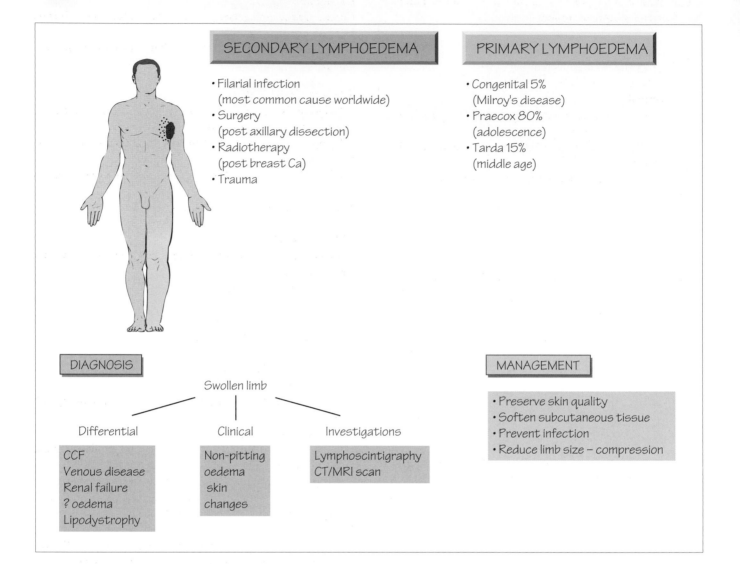

SECONDARY LYMPHOEDEMA

- Filarial infection
  (most common cause worldwide)
- Surgery
  (post axillary dissection)
- Radiotherapy
  (post breast Ca)
- Trauma

PRIMARY LYMPHOEDEMA

- Congenital 5%
  (Milroy's disease)
- Praecox 80%
  (adolescence)
- Tarda 15%
  (middle age)

DIAGNOSIS

Swollen limb

Differential

CCF
Venous disease
Renal failure
? oedema
Lipodystrophy

Clinical

Non-pitting
oedema
 skin
changes

Investigations

Lymphoscintigraphy
CT/MRI scan

MANAGEMENT

- Preserve skin quality
- Soften subcutaneous tissue
- Prevent infection
- Reduce limb size – compression

Definition

Lymphoedema is a persistent swelling of the tissues caused by the accumulation of protein-rich fluid as a result of failure of lymph transport from the tissues.

Key points

- Lymphoedema is a chronic condition that causes considerable morbidity.
- Filiariasis is the most common cause of lymphoedema worldwide.
- Up to 25% of patients post breast cancer therapy develop lymphoedema.
- Surgery is rarely indicated in the management of lymphoedema.

Classification of lymphoedema

Lymphoedema	Lymphatic defect
Primary (uncommon)	
Congenital (Milroy's disease) (rare)	Aplasia (15%)
Praecox—appears in adolescence (80% of primary lymphoedema)	Hypoplasia (70%)
Tarda—appears in middle age	Hyperplasia/ varicosity (15%)
Secondary (common)	
Infection (filiariasis,* TB, lymphogranuloma, actinomycosis, chronic lymphangitis	Hyperplastic/ varicose
Surgery (especially after axillary dissection for breast cancer)	
Radiation therapy (especially for breast cancer)	
Trauma	

* Parasitic infestation with filarial worm *Wuchereria bancrofti.*

Clinical features

Limb swelling

- Starts distally and ascends proximally over period of months.
- Characteristic 'tree trunk' appearance to lower limb.
- Absence of pigmentation differentiates lower limb lymphoedema from venous insufficiency.

Clinical grades

- Grade 1: pitting oedema and decrease in swelling on limb elevation.
- Grade 2: non-pitting oedema and little decrease in swelling on elevation.
- Grade 3 (elephantiasis): gross swelling of the limb with skin changes.

Investigations

- Diagnosis is usually made on history and clinical examination.
- (Lymphangiography)—not used anymore.
- Lymphoscintigraphy—best method of measuring lymphatic function.
- CT or MRI scanning of limb—good for imaging oedema and fibrosis.
- Duplex ultrasound to exclude venous disease.

Management

Lymphoedema is a chronic condition that cannot be cured but it can be managed.

Aims of management are to:
- Preserve skin quality.
- Soften subcutaneous tissue.
- Prevent lymphangitis.
- Reduce limb size.

Complex physical therapy:
- Complete decongestive therapy.
- Manual lymphatic drainage and exercise to promote lymph flow.
- Compression bandages.
- External pneumatic compression using sequential gradient pumps to decrease limb size.
- Compression sleeves and stockings to decrease limb size.
- Skin care to avoid infection and further lymphatic damage.
- Aggressive treatment of infection if it occurs.

Drug therapy:
- Flavonoids, antibiotics, diuretics (benzopyrones), (all have been used but usefulness unproven, benzopyrones may cause hepatic impairment).

Surgery (rarely indicated):
- Excisional debulking procedures (lymphangiectomy).
- Liposuction.
- Lymphatico-venous anastomosis.

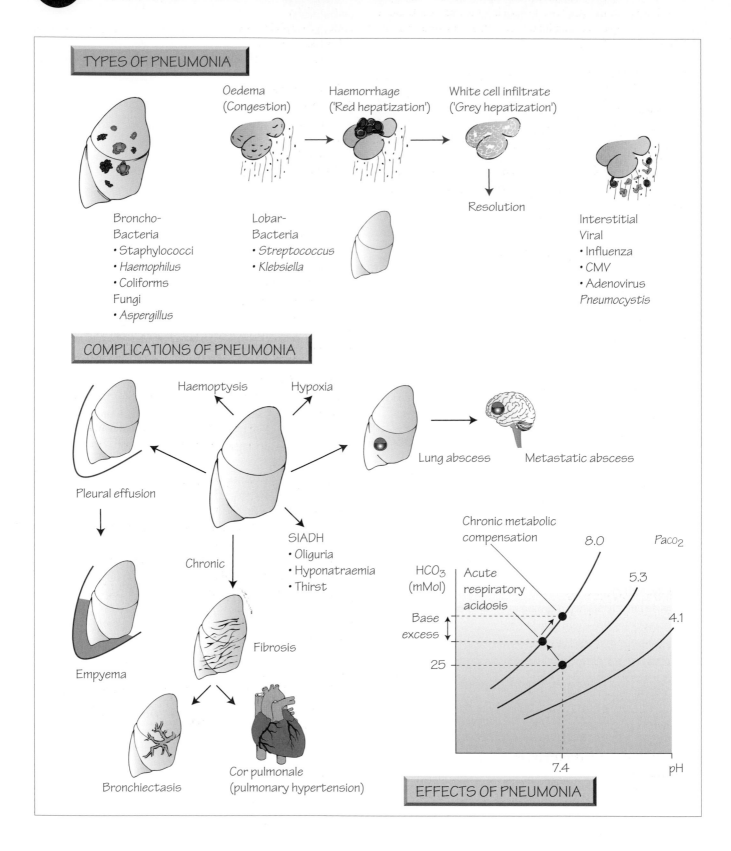

TYPES OF PNEUMONIA

Oedema (Congestion) → Haemorrhage ('Red hepatization') → White cell infiltrate ('Grey hepatization') → Resolution

Broncho-
Bacteria
• Staphylococci
• *Haemophilus*
• *Coliforms*
Fungi
• *Aspergillus*

Lobar-
Bacteria
• *Streptococcus*
• *Klebsiella*

Interstitial
Viral
• Influenza
• CMV
• Adenovirus
Pneumocystis

COMPLICATIONS OF PNEUMONIA

Haemoptysis   Hypoxia

Lung abscess   Metastatic abscess

Pleural effusion

SIADH
• Oliguria
• Hyponatraemia
• Thirst

Chronic

Fibrosis

Empyema

Bronchiectasis

Cor pulmonale (pulmonary hypertension)

EFFECTS OF PNEUMONIA

Chronic metabolic compensation

HCO_3 (mMol)

Acute respiratory acidosis

Pa_{CO_2}

8.0

5.3

4.1

Base excess

25

7.4   pH

Definitions

Pulmonary collapse or *atelectasis* results from alveolar hypoventilation such that the alveolar walls collapse and become de-aerated. *Pneumonia* is an infection with consolidation of the pulmonary parenchyma.

Key points

- Thoracic and upper abdominal incisions are at high risk of postoperative pulmonary collapse ± infection.
- Aggressive prophylaxis is key to prevention of complications.
- Postoperative pneumonia is often due to mixed organisms.
- Postoperative pulmonary complications prolong hospital stay by 1–2 weeks.

Aetiology/pathophysiology

Postoperatively patients frequently develop atelectasis, which may develop into a pneumonia.

Pulmonary collapse

- Proximal bronchial obstruction.
- Trapped alveolar air absorbed.
- Common in smokers.
- Common with COPD, asthma or sleep apnoea.

Pneumonia

- Infection with micro-organisms.
- Bacterial: *Streptococcus pneumoniae, Staphylococcus, Haemophilus influenzae*.
- Viral: influenza, CMV.
- Fungal: *Candida, Aspergillus*.
- Protozoal: *Pneumocystis, Toxoplasma*.

Pulmonary embolism

See venous thromboembolism (see Chapter 69).

Predisposing factors

- Secretional airway obstruction.
- Bronchorrhoea post surgery.
- Mucus plugs block bronchi.
- Impaired ciliary action.
- Postoperative pain prevents effective coughing (especially thoracotomy and upper laparotomies).
- Organic airway obstruction.
- Bronchial neoplasm.

Patients prone to severe pneumonia

- The elderly.
- Alcoholics.
- Chronic lung and heart disease.

- Debilitated patients.
- Diabetes.
- Post-CVA.
- Immunodeficiency states.
- Post-splenectomy.
- Atelectasis post surgery.

Clinical features

Pulmonary collapse

- Pyrexia.
- Tachypnoea.
- Diminished air entry.
- Bronchial breathing.

Pneumonia

- Respiratory distress.
- Painful dyspnoea.
- Tachypnoea.
- Productive cough ± haemoptysis.
- Hypoxia—confusion.
- Diminished air entry.
- Consolidation.
- Pleural rub.
- Cyanosis.

Investigations

- Chest X-ray: consolidation, pleural effusion, interstitial infiltrates, air–fluid cysts.
- Sputum culture: essential for correct antibiotic treatment.
- Blood gas analysis: diagnosis of respiratory failure.

Essential management

Prophylaxis

- Stop smoking—preferably for 8 weeks.
- Pre-operative deep-breathing exercises.
- Incentive spirometry and chest physiotherapy.
- Bronchodilators if needed.
- Adequate analgesia postoperatively.
- Early ambulation.

Treatment

- Pain control.
- Intensive chest physiotherapy.
- Respiratory support: humidified O_2 therapy; adequate hydration; bronchodilators if bronchospasm is present.
- Specific antimicrobial therapy.

Complications

- Respiratory failure.
- Lung abscess.

73 Bronchial carcinoma

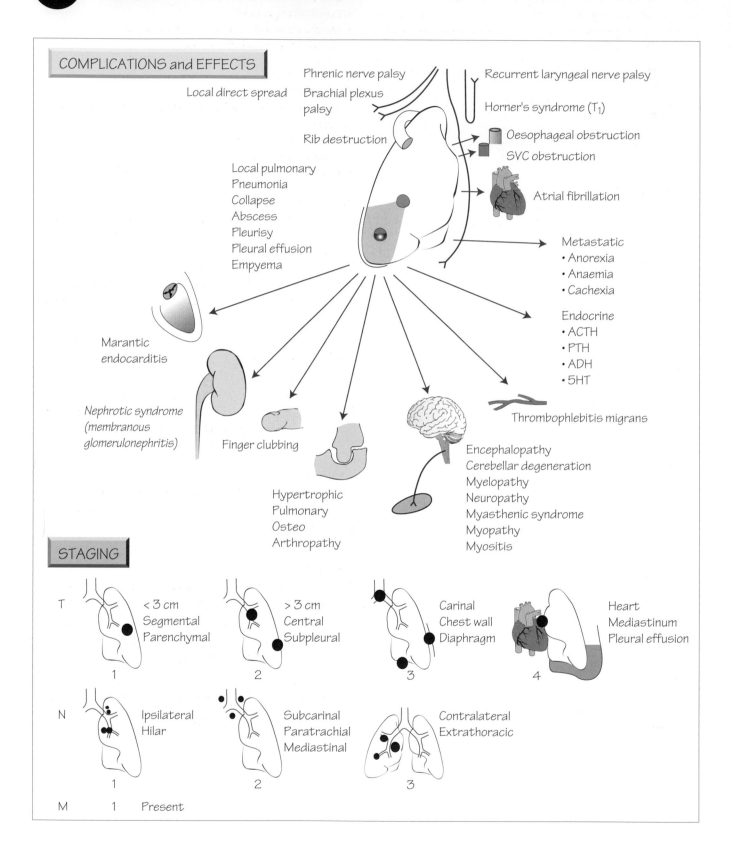

COMPLICATIONS and EFFECTS

Local direct spread

Phrenic nerve palsy

Brachial plexus palsy

Rib destruction

Recurrent laryngeal nerve palsy

Horner's syndrome (T_1)

Oesophageal obstruction

SVC obstruction

Atrial fibrillation

Local pulmonary
Pneumonia
Collapse
Abscess
Pleurisy
Pleural effusion
Empyema

Metastatic
• Anorexia
• Anaemia
• Cachexia

Endocrine
• ACTH
• PTH
• ADH
• 5HT

Marantic endocarditis

Nephrotic syndrome (membranous glomerulonephritis)

Finger clubbing

Hypertrophic Pulmonary Osteo Arthropathy

Thrombophlebitis migrans

Encephalopathy
Cerebellar degeneration
Myelopathy
Neuropathy
Myasthenic syndrome
Myopathy
Myositis

STAGING

T

1 < 3 cm
   Segmental
   Parenchymal

2 > 3 cm
   Central
   Subpleural

3 Carinal
   Chest wall
   Diaphragm

4 Heart
   Mediastinum
   Pleural effusion

N

1 Ipsilateral
   Hilar

2 Subcarinal
   Paratrachial
   Mediastinal

3 Contralateral
   Extrathoracic

M 1 Present

 Surgery at a Glance, 4e. By P. Grace and N.R. Borley. Published 2009 by Blackwell Publishing. ISBN 978-1-4051-8325-3.

Definition

Malignant lesion of the respiratory tree epithelium.

> ### Key points
>
> • Symptoms may be masked by coexistent lung pathology (COPD).
> • Bronchial carcinoma often presents late and most are non-resectable.
> • Surgically resectable tumours have a fair prognosis.

Epidemiology

Male : female 5 : 1. Uncommon before 50 years. Most patients are in their 60s. Accounts for 40 000 deaths per annum in the UK.

Aetiology

Predisposing factors:
• Cigarette smoking.
• Air pollution.
• Exposure to uranium, chromium, arsenic, haematite and asbestos.

Pathology

Histology

• Squamous carcinoma: 50%.
• Small-cell (oat-cell) carcinoma: 35%.
• Adenocarcinoma: 15%.

Spread

• Direct to pleura, recurrent laryngeal nerve, pericardium, oesophagus, brachial plexus.
• Lymphatic to mediastinal and cervical nodes.
• Haematogenous to liver, bone, brain, adrenals.
• Transcoelomic pleural seedlings and effusion.

Clinical features

• History of tiredness, cough, anorexia, weight loss.
• Productive cough with purulent sputum.
• Haemoptysis.
• Finger clubbing.
• Bronchopneumonia (secondary infection of collapsed lung segment distal to malignant bronchial obstruction).
• Pleuritic pain.
• Neuropathy, myopathy, hypertrophic osteoarthropathy.
• Endocrine syndromes (ACTH is secreted by oat-cell tumours, parathormone is secreted by SCC—hypercalcaemia).

• Pancoast's tumour (apical tumour invading sympathetic trunk and brachial plexus)—Horner's syndrome, brachial neuralgia, paralysis of upper limb.
• Dysphagia and broncho-oesophageal fistula.
• Superior vena caval obstruction.

Investigations

Diagnostic

• Chest X-ray—PA and lateral (lung opacity, hilar lymphadenopathy).
• CT-guided lung biopsy.
• Sputum cytology.
• Bronchoscopy and cytology of brushings or lavage fluid.

Assess operability

• Helical CT scan of thorax/abdomen: involvement of adjacent structures, hepatic metastases, multiple primary lesions.
• Bone scan: metastases.
• Liver ultrasound: metastases.
• Mediastinoscopy: involvement of mediastinal nodes.
• Lung function test: likely patient tolerance of pulmonary resection.

> ### Essential management
>
> #### Surgical
>
> • Indicated only for non-small cell tumours when tumour is confined to one lobe or lung, no evidence of secondary deposits, carina is tumour free on bronchoscopy.
> • Operation: lobectomy or pneumonectomy.
>
> #### Palliative
>
> Radiotherapy (small-cell carcinoma most radiosensitive): stop haemoptysis, relieve bone pain from secondaries, relieve SVC obstruction.

Prognosis

Following 'curative' resection 5-year survival rates are approximately 20–30%, but overall 5-year survival is only about 6%.

> ### 2 Week wait referral criteria for suspected lung cancer
>
> • CXR suspicious for malignancy.
> • Persistent haemoptysis in smoker or ex-smoker >40 years.
> • Signs of SVC obstruction.
> • Stridor.

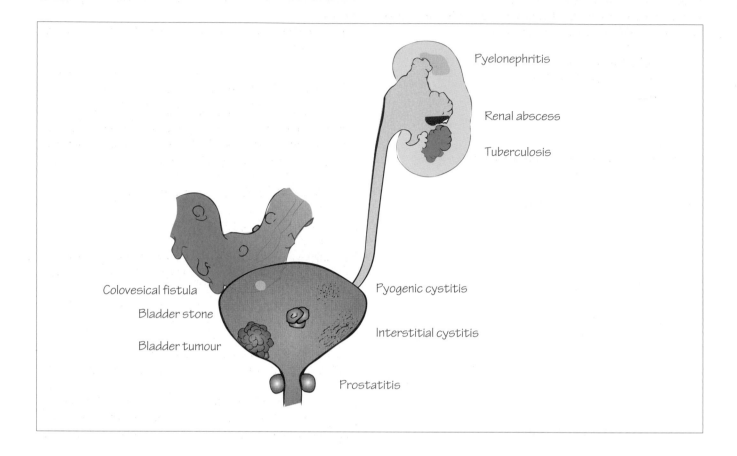

Pyelonephritis

Renal abscess

Tuberculosis

Pyogenic cystitis

Interstitial cystitis

Prostatitis

Colovesical fistula

Bladder stone

Bladder tumour

Definition

A *urinary tract infection* (UTI) is a documented episode of significant bacteriuria (i.e. an infection with a colony count of >100 000 single organisms per millilitre) which may affect the upper (*pyelonephritis*, *renal abscess*) or the lower (*cystitis*) urinary tract or both. *Colony forming units* (cfu; expressed as cfu/mL) represent the number of bacterial colonies per millilitre of sample.

Key points

• Lower UTI is usually harmless and simple to treat.
• Upper UTI may be associated with renal damage and major complications and requires prompt investigation and treatment.
• Consider an underlying cause in all recurrent or atypical infections.

Epidemiology

UTI is a very common condition in general practice (usually *Escherichia coli*) and accounts for 40% of hospital-acquired (*nosocomial*) infections (often *Enterobacter* or *Klebsiella*).

Risk factors

• Urinary tract obstruction.
• Instrumentation of urinary tract (e.g. indwelling catheter).
• Dysfunctional (neuropathic) bladder.
• Immunosuppression.
• Diabetes mellitus.
• Structural abnormalities (e.g. vesicoureteric reflux).
• Pregnancy.
• Dehydration

Pathology

- Ascending infection: most UTIs caused in this way (bacteria from GI tract colonize lower urinary tract).
- Haematogenous spread: infrequent cause of UTI (seen in IV drug users, bacterial endocarditis and TB).

Clinical features

Upper urinary tract infection

- Fever, rigors/chill.
- Flank pain.
- Malaise.
- Anorexia.
- Costovertebral angle and abdominal tenderness.
- May lead to septicaemia.

Lower urinary tract infection

- Dysuria.
- Frequency and urgency.
- Suprapubic pain.
- Haematuria.
- Scrotal pain (epididymo-orchitis) or perineal pain (prostatitis).

Investigations

Gram stain and culture of a 'clean-catch' urine specimen before antibiotics have been given. Usual organisms are *E. coli*, *Enterobacter*, *Klebsiella*, *Proteus* (suggests presence of urinary calculi). >100 000 single organism cfu/mL = infection, <100 000 cfu or mixed growth suggests contamination.

Upper urinary tract infection

- FBC.
- U+E and serum creatinine: renal function.
- Renal ultrasound: swelling in pyelonephritis, stones, obstruction/hydronephrosis, secondary abscess.
- IVU: stones, structural abnormalities, obstructed collecting system.
- CT scan: abscess/tumours.
- Renal scintigraphy or isotope scanning:
  ^{99m}Tc-MAG3 ± diuretic for assessing renal blood flow/function/obstruction
  ^{99m}Tc-DMSA for renal cortical assessment, e.g. cortical scarring

Lower urinary tract infection

- FBC.
- Cystoscopy only if haematuria—underlying neoplasm or stones.
- If obstruction is present ultrasound scan, IVU and cystoscopy may be needed.

Essential management

Treat the infection with an appropriate antibiotic based on urine culture results and deal with any underlying cause (e.g. relieve obstruction). High fluid intake should be encouraged and potassium citrate may relieve dysuria.

Upper tract UTIs, epididymo-orchitis and prostatitis

- IV antibiotic therapy (ciprofloxacin, gentamicin, cefuroxime, co-trimoxazole).
- Relieve acute obstruction with internal (double-J stent) or external (nephrostomy) drainage (especially if acute severe sepsis).
- An abscess will require drainage either radiologically or surgically.

Cystitis and uncomplicated lower UTI

- Oral antibiotics (trimethoprim, ciprofloxacin, nitrofurantoin, cefradine).
- If there is a poor response to treatment consider unusual urinary infections: tuberculosis (sterile pyuria), candiduria, schistosomiasis, *Chlamydia trachomatis*, *Neisseria gonorrhoeae*.
- Recurrent infections should raise the possibility of underlying abnormalities requiring investigation.

Complications

- Bacteraemia and septic shock.
- Renal, perinephric and metastatic abscesses.
- Renal damage and acute/chronic renal failure.
- Chronic and xanthogranulomatous pyelonephritis.

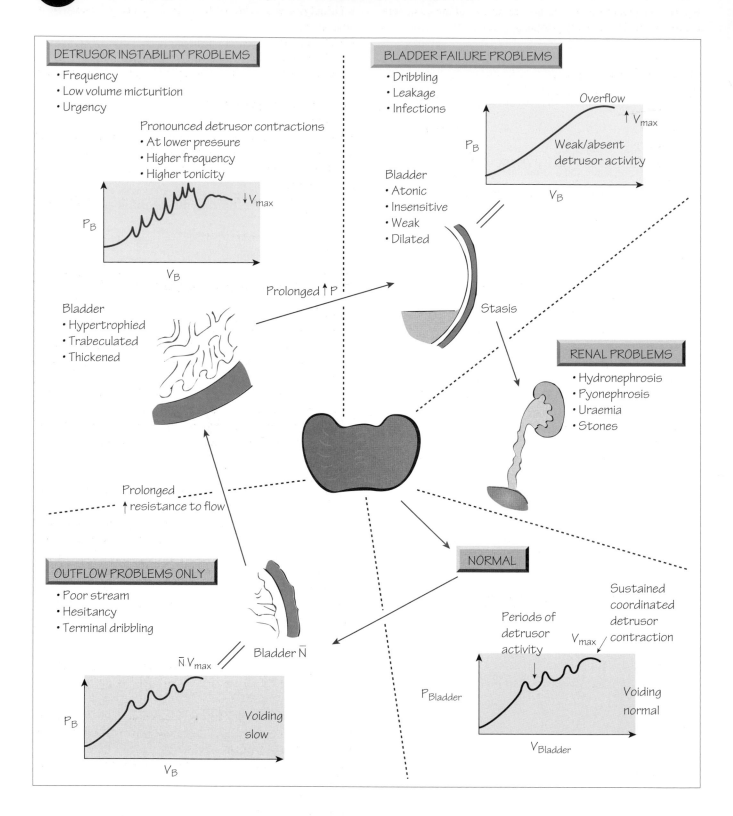

DETRUSOR INSTABILITY PROBLEMS

- Frequency
- Low volume micturition
- Urgency

Pronounced detrusor contractions
- At lower pressure
- Higher frequency
- Higher tonicity

$\downarrow V_{max}$

P_B

V_B

Bladder
- Hypertrophied
- Trabeculated
- Thickened

Prolonged $\uparrow P$

BLADDER FAILURE PROBLEMS

- Dribbling
- Leakage
- Infections

Overflow

$\uparrow V_{max}$

P_B

Weak/absent detrusor activity

V_B

Bladder
- Atonic
- Insensitive
- Weak
- Dilated

Stasis

RENAL PROBLEMS

- Hydronephrosis
- Pyonephrosis
- Uraemia
- Stones

Prolonged $\uparrow$ resistance to flow

OUTFLOW PROBLEMS ONLY

- Poor stream
- Hesitancy
- Terminal dribbling

$\bar{N} V_{max}$

Bladder $\bar{N}$

P_B

Voiding slow

V_B

NORMAL

Periods of detrusor activity

Sustained coordinated detrusor contraction

V_{max}

$P_{Bladder}$

Voiding normal

$V_{Bladder}$

Definition

Benign prostatic hypertrophy (BPH) is a condition of unknown aetiology characterized by an increase in size of the inner zone (periurethral glands) of the prostate gland.

Key points

- Symptoms of BPH are initially due to outflow problems, then bladder instability, then bladder failure.
- Obstruction-induced bladder dysfunction contributes significantly to symptoms.
- Early treatment of symptoms prevents/reverses bladder damage and complications.
- Surgical resection is safe but is associated with some significant complications.

Epidemiology

Present in 50% of 60–90-year-old men.

Pathophysiology

- Microscopic stromal nodules develop around the periurethral glands.
- Glandular hyperplasia originates around these nodules.
- As the gland increases in size, it compresses the urethra, leading to urinary tract obstruction and bladder dysfunction.

Clinical features

Initially outlet obstruction:

- Weak stream, hesitancy, intermittency, dribbling, straining to void, acute urinary retention.

Subsequent detrusor instability:

- Frequency, urgency, nocturia, dysuria, urge incontinence.

Finally detrusor failure and chronic retention:

- Palpable (or percussible) bladder, overflow incontinence.
- Enlarged smooth prostate on digital rectal examination.

Symptom score for BPH (International Prostate Symptom Score).

In past month	Never	<1 in 5 times	<50% of the time	50% of the time	>50% of the time	Almost always
Incomplete emptying	0	1	2	3	4	5
Frequency	0	1	2	3	4	5
Intermittency (stop and start)	0	1	2	3	4	5
Urgency	0	1	2	3	4	5
Weak stream	0	1	2	3	4	5
Straining	0	1	2	3	4	5
Nocturia	0	1	2	3	4	5

Total symptom score range 0–35.
0–7, mildly symptomatic; 8–19, moderately symptomatic; 20–35, severely symptomatic.

	Delighted	Mixed	Dissatisfied	Unhappy	Terrible
Bother score	0	1 2	3	4	5 6

Bother score gives an assessment of patient's perceived QoL.

Investigations

Basic investigations

- Urinalysis and urine culture for evidence of infection or haematuria.
- FBC: infection.
- U+E and serum creatinine: renal function.
- PSA: suspicion of underlying malignancy (very non-specific).

Further investigations

- Voiding diary.
- Uroflowmetry and post void residual volume measurement (normal <100 mL): evidence of obstruction.
- Ultrasonography of kidneys and bladder: structural abnormalities.
- TRUS: to determine prostate size/biopsy if malignancy suspected.
- IVU: structural abnormalities.
- Cystoscopy.

Essential management

Medical

- Alter oral fluid intake, reduce caffeine intake.
- Stop anticholinergic, sympathomimetic and opioid drugs.
- α-Adrenergic blockers (e.g. phenoxybenzamine, prazosin) to improve voiding.
- 5α-reductase inhibitors (e.g. finasteride) (cellular antiandrogens) to reduce prostate size.
- Intermittent self-catheterization if detrusor failure.
- Complete obstruction requires immediate catheterization.

Surgical

Most patients are treated surgically by removing the adenomatous part of the prostate by:

- TURP with electrocautery or laser for smaller prostates and open surgery (retropubic or suprapubic approach) for larger prostates (>75 g).
- Less invasive procedures include balloon dilatation, intraurethral stents, microwave or high-intensity focused ultrasound thermotherapy, laser ablation, electro- or radio-frequency vaporization.

Complications of surgical treatment

- Postoperative haemorrhage and clot retention.
- UTI.
- TURP syndrome: in 2% of patients absorption of irrigation fluid via venous sinuses in the prostate causes hyponatraemia, hypotension and metabolic acidosis.
- Erectile dysfunction (retrograde ejaculation, impotence) 5–35% of patients.
- Incontinence 1%.
- Urethral stricture.

Prognosis

The majority of patients have a very good QoL after prostatectomy (endoscopic or open).

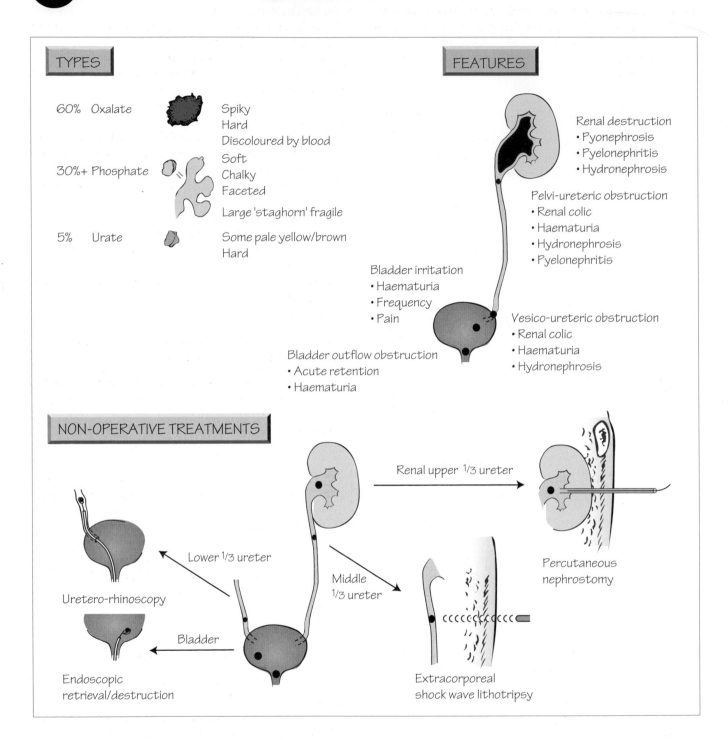

TYPES

60% Oxalate
Spiky
Hard
Discoloured by blood

30%+ Phosphate
Soft
Chalky
Faceted
Large 'staghorn' fragile

5% Urate
Some pale yellow/brown
Hard

FEATURES

Renal destruction
• Pyonephrosis
• Pyelonephritis
• Hydronephrosis

Pelvi-ureteric obstruction
• Renal colic
• Haematuria
• Hydronephrosis
• Pyelonephritis

Bladder irritation
• Haematuria
• Frequency
• Pain

Vesico-ureteric obstruction
• Renal colic
• Haematuria
• Hydronephrosis

Bladder outflow obstruction
• Acute retention
• Haematuria

NON-OPERATIVE TREATMENTS

Renal upper 1/3 ureter

Lower 1/3 ureter

Middle 1/3 ureter

Percutaneous nephrostomy

Uretero-rhinoscopy

Bladder

Endoscopic retrieval/destruction

Extracorporeal shock wave lithotripsy

Definition

Renal or *urinary* calculi are concretions formed by precipitation of various urinary solutes in the urinary tract. They contain calcium oxalate (60%), phosphate as a mixture of calcium, ammonium and magnesium phosphate—also called *struvite*—(triple phosphate stones are infective in origin) (30%), uric acid (5%) and cystine (1%).

Key points

- Calculi may develop because of or cause UTIs.
- Most stones (80–85%) pass without complication.
- Most stones are managed non-surgically.
- The pain of renal/ureteric calculi is very severe.
- Ureteric stone with obstruction and upper UTI is a urological emergency requiring immediate IV antibiotics and relief of the obstruction by ureteric stent or nephrostomy.
- Beware of the diagnosis of ureteric colic in patients >60 years—it might be a leaking AAA.

Epidemiology

Male : female 3 : 1. Early adult life. Among Europeans prevalence is 3%.

Pathogenesis

- Hypercalciuria: 65% of patients have idiopathic hypercalciuria.
- Nucleation theory: a crystal or foreign body acts as a nucleus for crystallization of supersaturated urine.
- Stone matrix theory: a protein matrix secreted by renal tubular cells acts as a scaffold for crystallization of supersaturated urine.
- Reduced inhibition theory: reduced urinary levels of naturally occurring inhibitors of crystallization.
- Dehydration.
- Infection: staghorn triple phosphate calculi are formed by the action of urease-producing organisms (*Proteus*, *Klebsiella*), which produce ammonia and render the urine alkaline.
- Schistosomiasis predisposes to bladder calculi (and cancer).

Pathology

- Staghorn calculi are large, fill the renal pelvis and calices, and lead to recurring pyelonephritis and renal parenchymal damage.
- Other stones are smaller, ranging in size from a few millimetres to 1–2 cm. They cause problems by obstructing the urinary tract, usually the ureter. Calyceal stones may cause haematuria and bladder stones may cause infection. Chronic bladder stones predispose to squamous carcinoma of the bladder (rare).

Clinical features

- Calyceal stones may be asymptomatic.
- Staghorn calculi present with loin pain and upper UTI.
- Ureteric colic—severe colicky pain radiating from the loin to the groin and into the testes or labia associated with gross or microscopic haematuria.
- Bladder calculi present with sudden interruption of urinary stream, perineal pain and pain at the tip of the penis.

Investigations

- FBC, U+E, serum creatinine, calcium, phosphate, urate, proteins and alkaline phosphatase.
- Urine microscopy for haematuria (present in most patients with urinary calculi) and crystals.
- Urine culture: secondary infection.
- Urine pH: <5.0 suggests uric acid stones, >7.0 suggests urea splitting organisms.
- Kidney, ureter, bladder (KUB) radiograph: 90% of renal calculi are radio-opaque.
- CT scanning: non-contrast helical CT scanning is more accurate than IVU in detecting urinary tract calculi. Gives no information about degree of obstruction or renal function.
- IVU: confirms the presence and the position of the stone in the genitourinary tract.
- An ultrasound may be indicated to exclude AAA. May show hydronephrosis or hydroureter if obstruction present.
- A renogram: may be indicated with staghorn calculi to assess renal function.
- 24-hour urine collection when patient is at home in normal environment.
- Stone analysis: origin.

Essential management

- Pain relief for ureteric colic: pethidine, diclofenac (NSAIDs as effective as opoids).
- High fluid intake.
- Antiemetics if required
- Oral α-adrenergic blockers increase rate of spontaneous stone passage.
- 80–85% of ureteric stones pass spontaneously. Stones of <4 mm in diameter almost always pass, >6 mm almost never pass.
- Indications for intervention:
  kidney stones: symptomatic, obstruction, staghorn
  ureteric stones: failure to pass, large stone, obstruction, infection
  bladder stones: all to prevent complications
  sepsis super-added: nephrostomy.

Interventional procedures

- ESWL for small/medium kidney stones.
- Percutaneous nephrolithotomy for large kidney stones and staghorn calculi.
- Ureteroscopy and manipulation of stone back into renal pelvis for ESWL or contact lithotrypsy for upper ureteric stones (above pelvic brim).
- Ureteroscopy with contact lithotripsy or extraction with a Dormia basket for lower ureteric stones.
- Open surgery: ureterolithotomy (rare now) or nephrolithotomy.
- Mechanical lithotripsy or open surgery for bladder stones.

77

Renal cell carcinoma

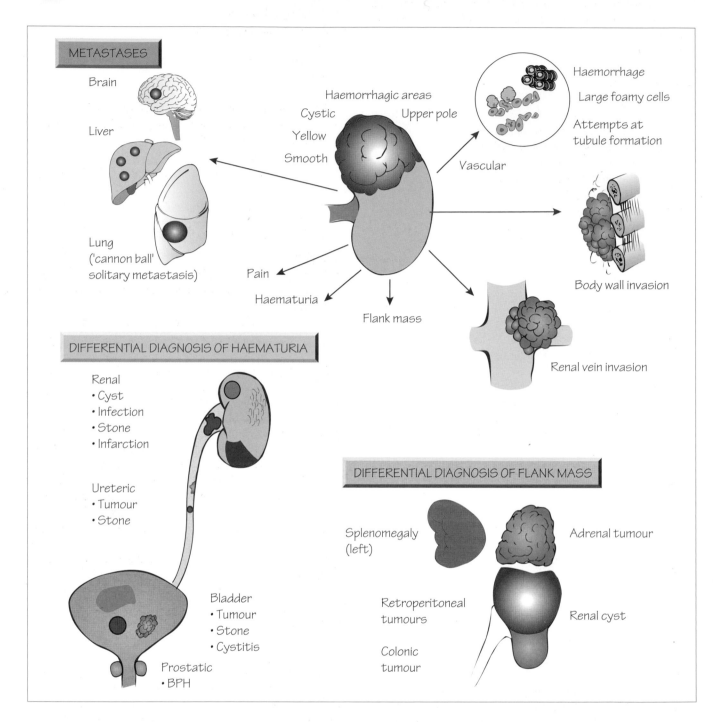

Definition

Malignant lesion (*adenocarcinoma*) of the kidney arising from the proximal renal tubular epithelium (also known as *hypernephroma* and *Grawitz' tumour*).

Key points

• New, significant haematuria always requires investigation and may represent renal cell carcinoma (RCC).

• Consider RCC in unexplained anaemia, vague abdominal symptoms and recurrent UTIs. RCC is one of the great 'mimics' of medicine.
• Surgery offers the best hope of long-term survival.
• Tumours are occasionally familial and a family history should be sought.

Epidemiology

Male : female 1.6 : 1. Uncommon before 40 years. Accounts for 2–3% of all tumours in adults and 85% of all renal tumours. (Other renal tumours: urothelial tumours, Wilms' tumour and sarcomas.)

Aetiology

Predisposing factors

- Diet: high intake of fat, oil and milk.
- Toxic agents: lead, cadmium, asbestos, petroleum byproducts, large amounts of phenacetin-containing analgesics.
- Cigarette smoking doubles the risk of RCC.
- Obesity especially in women.
- Genetic factors: oncogene on short arm of chromosome 3, HLA antigen BW-44 and DR-8.
- Other diseases: von Hippel–Lindau (VHL) syndrome, hereditary papillary renal carcinoma, adult polycystic disease, renal dialysis patients, post-renal transplantation.

Pathology

Histology

Adenocarcinoma (cell of origin is the proximal renal tubular epitheliuml). Histological subtypes are: clear cell (75%), chromophilic (15%), chromophobic (5%), oncocytoma (3%—rarely metastasize) and collecting duct (2%—very aggressive).

Spread

- Direct into renal vein and perirenal tissue.
- Lymphatic to periaortic and hilar nodes.
- Haematogenous to lung (large, 'cannon-ball' metastases), bones and contralateral kidney.

Staging

TNM staging.

Robson stages I–IV	5-year survival
Stage I: tumour confined within renal capsule	66%
Stage II: tumour confined by Gerota's fascia	64%
Stage III: tumour to renal vein or IVC, nodes or through Gerota's fascia	42%
Stage IV: distant metastases or invasion of adjacent organs	11%

Clinical features

- Triad of haematuria (40–60%), flank pain (40–50%), abdominal mass (25–45%) but all three in <10% of patients.
- Hypertension (20%), polycythaemia (due to decreased blood flow to JGA → $\uparrow$ renin, $\uparrow$ erythropoietin).
- Anaemia, weight loss, PUO, night sweats, malaise.
- Paraneoplastic conditions (caused by tumour release of IL-6, erythropoietin or nitric oxide):
  hypercalcaemia, ectopic hormone production (ACTH, ADH)
  liver dysfunction (raised enzymes and prolonged PT) in the absence of metastatic disease (Stauffer's syndrome)
  polyneuropathy, myopathy, cachexia, dermatomyositis
- Left-sided varicocele (2% of males with RCC).

- 30% present with metastatic disease (lung, soft tissues, bone, liver, skin, CNS).

Investigations

- FBC: anaemia, polycythaemia.
- ESR.
- U+E, calcium, creatinine: renal function.
- LFTs: metastases.
- Urine culture: infection.
- Abdominal ultrasound: assess renal mass and IVC.
- Contrast-enhanced CT scan: imaging modality of choice for diagnosis and staging of RCC.
- IVU: image renal outline.
- MRA, cavagram and echocardiogram: assess IVC and right atrium involvement.
- Bone scan if bony symptoms and raised alkaline phosphatase.

Essential management

Surgical

- Young patients—offers best chance of long-term survival.
- Elderly patients—life expectancy may be short (= to that with supportive treatment only).
- Radical (laparoscopic) nephrectomy: aim to remove kidney, renal vessels, upper ureter, (± ipsilateral adrenal gland) and Gerota's fascia.
- Partial nephrectomy: if Stage I and part of VHL presentation.
- Isolated lung/brain metastases may also be removed surgically with good results.

Palliative

- Palliative surgery (nephrectomy) considered pain, haemorrhage, malaise, hypercalcaemia or polycythaemia.
- Multikinase inhibitors (e.g. sorafenib, sunitinib) induce partial response in 40% of patients with advanced disease and prolong survival by 6–9 months. May be toxic side-effects.
- Chemotherapy (only 10% response rate)—no standard regimen.
- Hormone therapy (only 5% response rate)—no standard regimen.
- Immunotherapy (IL-2, interferon, BCG—selected patients will respond).
- Radiotherapy for local or metastatic symptoms.

Prognosis

50% of early stage RCCs are cured but outcome for Stage IV is very poor. Overall survival is 40% at 5 years.

2 Week wait referral criteria for suspected urological cancer

- Macroscopic haematuria in adult.
- Microscopic haematuria >50 years.
- Testicular body swelling.
- Solid renal mass on imaging.
- Increased PSA (if life expectancy >10 years).
- Increased PSA with malignant feeling prostate/bone pain.
- Suspected penile cancer.

78

Carcinoma of the bladder

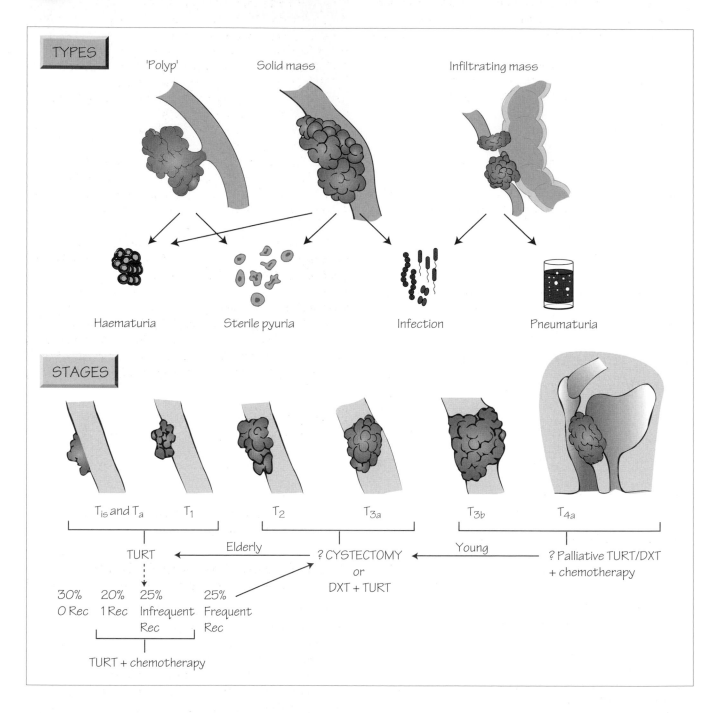

Definition

Malignant lesion of the bladder epithelium.

Key points

- Commonly presents with haematuria.
- Ranges from 'benign' acting recurrent bladder 'polyps' to rapidly progressive infiltrating masses.
- Transitional cell lesions are a 'field' change and often multiple.

Epidemiology

Male : female 3 : 1. Uncommon before 50 years. Increasing incidence of bladder cancer in recent years. Death rate is 7.6/100 000.

Aetiology

Predisposing factors:

- Smoking is associated with 50% of all bladder cancers. Carcinogens in smoke include 2-naphthylamine, 4-aminobiphenyl and nitrosamines.
- Exposure to aromatic amines in dyes, paints, solvents and rubber.

- Prior exposure to radiation of the pelvis or chemotherapy with cyclophosphamide (via exposure to its metabolite, acrolein).
- Bladder irritation from *Schistosomiasis*, bladder stones or long-term indwelling catheters (squamous carcinoma).
- Congenital abnormalities (extrophy of the bladder) (adenocarcinoma).
- Genetic mutations of tumour suppressor genes on chromosomes 17 (*p53*, high grade) and 9 (*p15* and *p16*, low grade) are linked to bladder cancer. Other mutations may also be involved.

Pathology
Histology
- Transitional cell carcinoma (TCC) or urothelial carcinoma (90%).
- Squamous cell carcinoma (5%). (In developing world SCC is common because of association with *Schistosomiasis*).
- Adenocarcinoma (2%).

Staging for TCC

(10%)	T_{CIS}	Carcinoma *in situ*
Superficial tumours (70%)	T_a	Tumour confined to urothelium
	T_1	Lamina propria involved
Invasive tumours (25%)	T_2	Muscularis propria invasion
	T_3	Perivesical fat invasion
Advanced tumours (5%)	T_4	Invasion of adjacent pelvic organs

N+ lymph node metastases, M+ distant metastases.

Spread
- Direct into pelvic viscera (prostate, uterus, vagina, colon, rectum).
- Lymphatic to periaortic nodes.
- Haematogenous to liver and lung.

Clinical features
- Painless intermittent gross haematuria (95%).
- Dysuria, urgency or frequency (10%).

Investigations
- Urine cytology (significant false negative rate).
- CT urography or IVU: occult upper tract tumours.
- Cystourethroscopy and biopsy.
- FBC: anaemia.
- U+E creatinine: renal function.
- Ultrasound: obstruction.
- CT scan: local invasion, distant metastases.

Essential management
Superficial tumours (T_{CIS}, T_a, T_1)
- TURT of bladder and surveillance cystoscopy.
- Intravesical immunotherapy with BCG ± interferon-α or interferon-γ. Patients with recurrence of T_{CIS} after BCG should be considered for radical cystectomy as most (80%) will progress to muscle invasive bladder cancer.
- Intravesical chemotherapy may be useful in patients refractory to intravesical immunotherapy.

Invasive tumours (T_2, T_3)
- Cystoprostatectomy (men) or anterior pelvic enenteration (women) + pelvic lymphadenectomy + urinary diversion (e.g. ileal conduit) (± adjuvant or neoadjuvant chemotherapy – controversial, not proven). 90% 5-year survival if tumour confined to bladder.
- External beam radiation therapy has been used but results not as good as radical surgery—20–40% 5-year survival if tumour confined to bladder.

Metastatic disease
- Chemotherapy: (MVAC) methotrexate, vinblastine, doxorubicin (Adriamycin), cisplatin or (GC) gemcitabine and cisplatin, (CMV) cisplatin, methotrexate, vinblastine. Most patients will die within 2 years in spite of Rx.

Prognosis
- Superficial tumours: 80–100% 5-year survival.
- Invasive tumours:
  T_2 70% 5-year survival
  T_3 50% 5-year survival
  T_4 10% 5-year survival
- Fixed tumours and metastases: median survival 1 year.
- Long-term follow-up required for life.

2 Week wait referral criteria for suspected urological cancer

- Macroscopic haematuria in adult.
- Microscopic haematuria >50 years.
- Testicular body swelling.
- Solid renal mass on imaging.
- Increased PSA (if life expectancy >10 years).
- Increased PSA with malignant feeling prostate/bone pain.
- Suspected penile cancer.

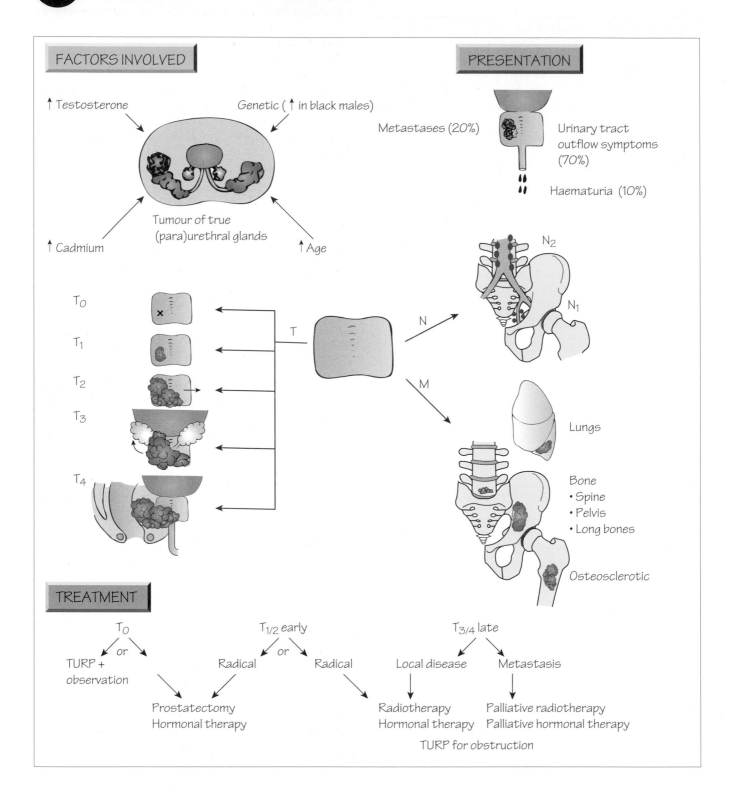

FACTORS INVOLVED

↑ Testosterone

Genetic (↑ in black males)

↑ Cadmium

Tumour of true
(para)urethral glands

↑ Age

T_0

T_1

T_2

T_3

T_4

T

N

M

PRESENTATION

Metastases (20%)

Urinary tract
outflow symptoms
(70%)

Haematuria (10%)

N_2

N_1

Lungs

Bone
• Spine
• Pelvis
• Long bones

Osteosclerotic

TREATMENT

T_0

or

TURP +
observation

$T_{1/2}$ early

or

Radical

Radical

Prostatectomy
Hormonal therapy

$T_{3/4}$ late

Local disease

Metastasis

Radiotherapy
Hormonal therapy

Palliative radiotherapy
Palliative hormonal therapy

TURP for obstruction

Definition

Malignant lesion of the prostate gland.

Key points

- Prostatic cancer is common and should be considered in all new symptoms of lower urinary tract obstruction.
- Increasingly found (asymptomatic) by screening using PSA and digital rectal examination. Need prostatic biopsy to make diagnosis.
- Early treatment offers good 5-year survival with combined surgery and hormonal adjuvants.
- Late presentation disease is best managed medically and has a poor outlook.

Epidemiology

Uncommon before 60 years. 80% of prostate cancers are clinically undetected (latent carcinoma) and are only discovered on autopsy. The true incidence of this disease is considerably higher than the clinical experience would indicate.

Aetiology

- Increasing age.
- More common in black men.
- Hormonal factors: prostate cancer growth is enhanced by testosterone and inhibited by oestrogens or antiandrogens.

Pathology

Prostatic tumours are often multicentric and located in the periphery of the gland.

Histology

- Adenocarcinoma arising from glandular epithelium.
- Gleason grading (1–5) is used to grade differentiation. The most common and second most common pattern are each graded 1–5; the sum of these gives the Gleason score (2–10).

Staging

	T_0	Unsuspected
Localized	T_1	Histological diagnosis only (clinical, radiology negative)
	T_2	Palpable—confined within prostate
Local spread	T_3	Spread to seminal vesicles
	T_4, N_1	Spread to pelvic wall
Metastatic	T_{1-4}, M_1	Metastatic disease

Spread

- Direct into remainder of gland and seminal vesicles.
- Lymphatic to iliac and periaortic nodes.
- Haematogenous to bone (usually osteosclerotic lesions), liver, lung.

Clinical features

- Bladder outflow obstruction (poor stream, hesitancy, nocturia).
- Symptoms of advanced disease (ureteric obstruction and hydronephrosis or bone pain from metastases, classically worse at night).
- Nodule or irregular firm mass detected on rectal examination.

Investigations

- FBC: anaemia.
- U+E, creatinine: renal function.
- Specific markers: PSA, PSA velocity (three measurements over 2 years), free : total PSA ratio.
- Transrectal U/S and MRI: local staging.
- Transrectal U/S guided needle biopsy of the prostate: tissue diagnosis.
- Bone scan: metastases.

Essential management

Localized prostate cancer

Risk	PSA (ng/mL)		Gleason		Clinical	Rx
Low	<10	+	≤6	+	T1–T2a	Active surveillance
Intermediate	10–20	or	7	or	T2b–T2c	Radical
High	>20	or	8–10	or	T3–T4	Radical

Active surveillance: observed for biochemical, histological or clinical progression. If progression occurs patients should be offered radical Rx.

Radical: radical prostatectomy or radiotherapy (external beam or brachytherapy).

Locally advanced prostate cancer (T3a–T4)

Radical radiotherapy ± neoadjuvant LHRHa + adjuvant hormonal therapy.

Metastatic prostate cancer

Hormonal therapy (bilateral orchidectomy, antiandrogen monotherapy [bicalutamide]).

For hormone-resistant cancers—docetaxel, steroids, strontium-89 for painful bone metastases.

Prognosis

- Localized tumours: 80% 5-year survival.
- Local spread: 40% 5-year survival.
- Metastases: 20% 5-year survival.

2 Week wait referral criteria for suspected urological cancer

- Macroscopic haematuria in adult.
- Microscopic haematuria >50 years.
- Testicular body swelling.
- Solid renal mass on imaging.
- Increased PSA (if life expectancy >10 years).
- Increased PSA with malignant feeling prostate/bone pain.
- Suspected penile cancer.

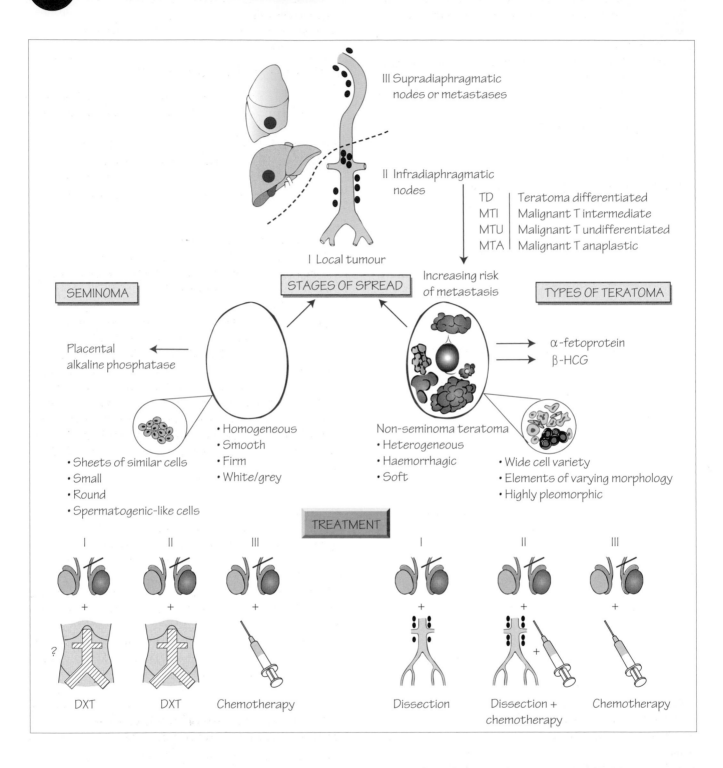

Definition

Malignant lesion of the testis.

Key points

• All newly discovered testicular lumps require investigation to exclude malignancy.

• Early tumours have an excellent prognosis with surgery alone.
• Late tumours have a good prognosis with surgery and medical therapy.
• Orchidectomy for tumour should be via a groin incision.
• Prognosis is generally good but depends on stage and histology.

Epidemiology

Age 20–35 years. Most common solid tumours in young males. The incidence of testicular cancer seems to be increasing.

Aetiology

- Crypto-orchidism—50-fold increase in risk of developing testicular germ cell cancer. Risk is unaffected by orchidopexy.
- Exposure to high prenatal oestrogen levels, chemical carcinogens, trauma, orchitis.
- Higher incidence in white men.

Pathology

Classification of testicular tumours

- Germ-cell tumours (95%) (secrete AFP and β-HCG):
  seminoma (SGCT) (40%)
  non-seminoma (NSGCT)—embryonal carcinoma (25%), teratoma/teratocarcinoma (30%), choriocarcinoma (1%), yolk sac tumour (rare)
- Non-germ-cell tumours (stromal tumours) (5%):
  Leydig cell
  Sertoli cell
  granulosa cell
  These are rare tumours and only 10% of them are malignant.
- Metastatic tumours.

Staging

- Stage I: confined to scrotum.
- Stage II: spread to retroperitoneal lymph nodes (IIa, nodes <2 cm; IIb, 2–5 cm; IIc, >5 cm) below the diaphragm.
- Stage III: distant metastases.

Spread

- Germ-cell tumours to para-aortic nodes, lung and brain.
- Stromal tumours rarely metastasize.

Clinical features

- Painless, hard swelling of the testis, often discovered incidentally or after trauma.
- Vague testicular discomfort common, bleeding into tumour may mimic acute torsion.
- Rarely evidence of metastatic disease or gynaecomastia (5%).
- Examination: hard, irregular, non-tender testicular mass.

Investigations

- Blood for tumour markers, i.e. AFP, β-HCG and LDH. Very useful in following success of treatment.
- AFP is elevated in 75% of embryonal and 65% of teratocarcinoma.
- AFP is *not* elevated in pure seminoma or choriocarcinoma. If an AFP elevation is noted in a pathologically diagnosed seminoma, the diagnosis should be changed to NSGCT.
- β-HCG is elevated in 100% choriocarcinoma, 60% embryonal carcinoma, 60% teratocarcinoma and 10% pure seminoma.
- Scrotal ultrasound: diagnosis is made by seeing a mass in the testis usually confined by the tunica albuginea.
- Chest X-ray to assess lungs and mediastinum: metastases.
- CT scan of chest and abdomen and pelvis: to detect lymph nodes and stage disease.
- Consider sperm banking for future fertility options.

Essential management

Radical orchidectomy (via groin incision) and histological diagnosis. Further treatment depends on histology and staging.

Seminoma

- Stage I: external beam radiotherapy to abdominal nodes.
- Stage II: external beam radiotherapy to abdominal nodes.
- Stage III: chemotherapy (bleomycin, etoposide, cisplatin [BEP]).

Non-seminoma germ cell

- Stage I: options (>90% cure with all options):
  aggressive surveillance and RPLND ± platinum-based chemotherapy if recurrence, or
  primary RPLND, or
  primary platinum-based chemotherapy (e.g. BEP).
- Stage II: platinum-based chemotherapy + RPLND.
- Stage III: primary chemotherapy (+ RPLND if good response). Stage III can be subdivided into good, intermediate and poor risk, depending on levels of tumour markers, size of mediastinal nodes, presence of cervical nodes and number of mediastinal metastases. (RPLND may be complicated by lack of antegarde ejaculation. RLPND may be performed laparoscopically with good results and less morbidity than the open approach.)

Prognosis

- Overall cure rates for testicular cancer are over 90% and node-negative disease has almost 100% 5-year survival.
- SGCT: Stage I and II, 98–100% 5-year survival; Stage III, 86–90% 5-year survival.
- NSGCT: Stage I, 98% 5-year survival; Stage II, 92% 5-year survival; Stage III, good risk 92%, intermediate risk 80% and poor risk 48% 5-year survival.
- Survivors of testicular cancer are at a significantly increased risk of secondary cancers because of young age and exposure to radiotherapy and/or chemotherapy.

---

2 Week wait referral criteria for suspected urological cancer

- Macroscopic haematuria in adult.
- Microscopic haematuria >50 years.
- Testicular body swelling.
- Solid renal mass on imaging.
- Increased PSA (if life expectancy >10 years).
- Increased PSA with malignant feeling prostate/bone pain.
- Suspected penile cancer.

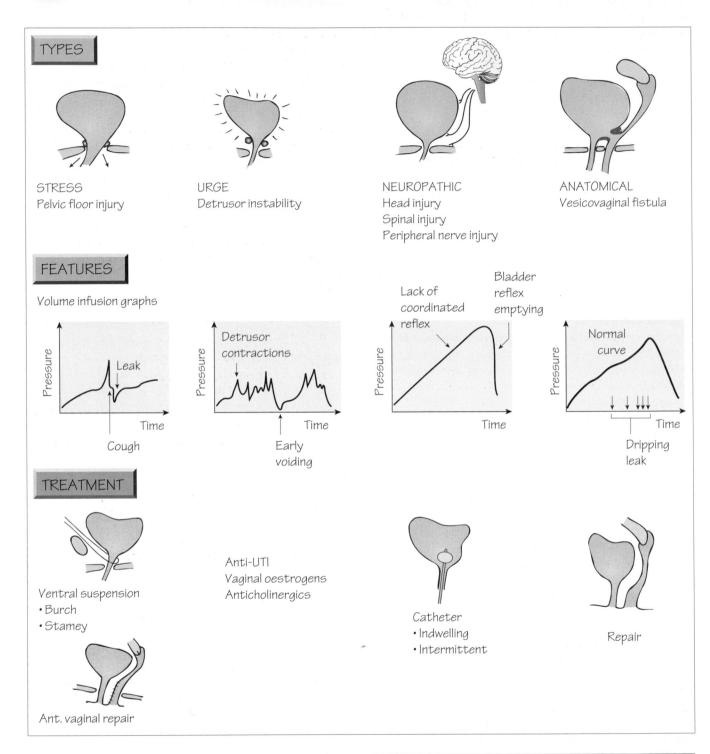

TYPES

STRESS
Pelvic floor injury

URGE
Detrusor instability

NEUROPATHIC
Head injury
Spinal injury
Peripheral nerve injury

ANATOMICAL
Vesicovaginal fistula

FEATURES

Volume infusion graphs

Leak
Cough

Detrusor contractions
Early voiding

Lack of coordinated reflex
Bladder reflex emptying

Normal curve
Dripping leak

TREATMENT

Ventral suspension
• Burch
• Stamey

Ant. vaginal repair

Anti-UTI
Vaginal oestrogens
Anticholinergics

Catheter
• Indwelling
• Intermittent

Repair

Definition

Urinary incontinence (UI) is defined as the involuntary loss of urine that can be demonstrated objectively and is a social or hygienic problem.

Key points

• A common and socially disabling condition.
• Full assessment and investigation is required to elicit precise cause and tailor treatment properly.
• Always assess if bladder full or empty (overflow or otherwise).

Epidemiology

UI affects 15–30% of the general population. More common in females (male : female 3 : 1) and in the elderly. UI rarely causes death but is a huge source of morbidity (perineal irritation and sepsis, frequency and nocturia, social isolation and embarrassment).

Classification

Urethral incontinence

• Urethral abnormalities: obesity, multiparity, difficult delivery, pelvic fractures, post-prostatectomy.
• Bladder abnormalities: neuropathic or non-neuropathic detrusor abnormalities, infection, interstitial cystitis, bladder stones and tumours.
• Non-urinary abnormalities: impaired mobility or mental function.

Non-urethral incontinence

• Urinary fistula: vesicovaginal.
• Ureteral ectopia: ureter drains into urethra (usually a duplex ureter).

Pathophysiology

• *Stress incontinence*: urine leakage when infra-abdominal pressure exceeds urethral pressure (e.g. coughing, laughing, straining or lifting). Urethral incompetence often develops as a result of impaired urethral support due to pelvic floor muscle weakness.
• *Urge incontinence*: uninhibited bladder contraction from detrusor hyperactivity causes a rise in intravesical pressure and urine leakage. May be caused by loss of cortical control (e.g. stroke) or bladder inflammation from stone, infection or neoplasm. Characterized by an overactive bladder: urgency, frequency and nocturia.
• *Mixed incontinence* is a combination of stress and urge incontinence.
• *Overflow incontinence*: damage to the efferent fibres of the sacral reflex causes bladder atonia. The bladder fills with urine and becomes grossly distended with constant dribbling of urine. May result from bladder outlet obstruction (e.g. BPH), spinal cord injury or congenital defect (e.g. spina bifida) or neuropathy (e.g. diabetes).

Clinical features

• Stress incontinence: loss of urine during coughing, straining, etc. These symptoms are quite specific for stress incontinence.
• Urge incontinence: inability to maintain urine continence in the presence of frequent and insistent urges to void.
• Nocturnal enuresis: 10% of 5-year-olds and 5% of 10-year-olds are incontinent during sleep. Bed-wetting in older children is abnormal and may indicate the presence of an unstable bladder.
• If symptoms of infection (frequency, dysuria, nocturia), obstruction (poor stream, dribbling), trauma (including surgery,

e.g. abdominoperineal resection), fistula (continuous dribbling), neurological disease (sexual or bowel dysfunction) or systemic disease (e.g. diabetes) an underlying cause.

Investigations

• Urine culture: to exclude infection.
• IVU: to assess upper tracts and obstruction or fistula.
• Urodynamics—essential in determining type of incontinence accurately:
  uroflowmetry: measures flow rate
  cystometry: demonstrates detrusor contractures
  video cystometry: shows leakage of urine on straining in patients with stress incontinence
  urethral pressure flowmetry: measures urethral and bladder pressure at rest and during voiding
  postvoid residual volume is measured by passing a catheter and draining the bladder 5 minutes after micturition.
• Cystoscopy: if bladder stone or neoplasm is suspected.
• Vaginal speculum examination ± cystogram if vesicovaginal fistula suspected.
• MRI to visualize pelvic floor defects.

Essential management

Urge incontinence

• Medical treatment: modify fluid intake, avoid caffeine and alcohol, treat any underlying cause (infection, tumour, stone); bladder training; anticholinergics/smooth muscle relaxants (oxybutynin, tolterodine).
• Surgical treatment (uncommon): cystoscopy and bladder distension, augmentation cystoplasty.

Stress incontinence

• Medical treatment: lose weight, pelvic floor exercises, oestrogens for atrophic vaginitis.
• Surgical treatment (common): retropubic or endoscopic urethropexy, vaginal repair, artificial sphincter, periurethral bulking injections.

Overflow incontinence

• Avoid medicines that cause detrusor hypoactivity: anticholinergics, calcium-channel blockers.
• If obstruction present: treat cause of obstruction, e.g. TURP.
• If no obstruction: short period of catheter drainage to allow detrusor muscle to recover from over-stretching, then short course of detrusor muscle stimulants (bethanechol; distigmine). Clean intermittent self-catheterization is a very effective way to manage neurogenic overflow incontinence.

Urinary fistula

• Always requires surgical treatment.

RENAL

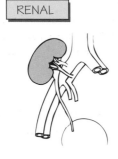

Typical outcomes
1 yr graft survival 90%
5 yr graft survival 65%

- Typical indications
  - Diabetic nephropathy
  - Glomerulopathies
  - Renal cystic disease
  - Renal arterial disease
  - Metabolic diseases
- Technical notes
  - Donor sources (cadaveric, LRD, LURD)
  - Graft placed in iliac fossa
  - Blood supply from external iliac vessels
  - Ureter implanted into bladder
- Typical complications
  - Acute rejection
  - Chronic rejection
  - Urine leak ('urinoma')
  - Vascular thrombosis
  - Lymphatic leak ('lymphocoele')

HEPATIC

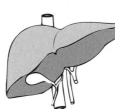

Typical outcomes
1 yr graft survival 80%
5 yr graft survival 55%

- Typical indications
  - Alcoholic disease
  - Viral hepatitis
  - Toxin induced liver failure
  - Autoimmune hepatic/biliary diseases
  - Metabolic diseases
  - Congenital disorders
  - Budd–Chiari syndrome
- Technical notes
  - Donor sources (cadaveric, LRD, LURD)
  - May be part of a liver or complete liver
- Typical complications
  - Primary acute non-function
  - Bile leak
  - Recurrent coronary artery disease
  - Vascular thrombosis
  - Biliary stricture

LUNG

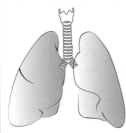

Typical outcomes
1 yr graft survival 70%
5 yr graft survival 55%

- Typical indications
  - COPD
  - Cystic fibrosis
  - Fibrosing alveolitides
  - Pulmonary hypertension
- Technical notes
  - Donor sources (cadaveric, LURD ('domino'))
  - May be part combined heart–lung, double lung or single lung
- Typical complications
  - Pulmonary infection

CARDIAC

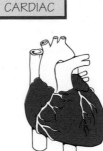

Typical outcomes
1 yr graft survival 80%
5 yr graft survival 65%

- Typical indications
  - Cardiomyopathies
  - Ischaemic heart disease
  - Congenital heart disease
- Technical notes
  - Donor sources (cadaveric)
  - Fully anatomical transplantation
- Typical complications
  - Acute rejection
  - Chronic rejection
  - Recurrent coronary artery disease

PANCREATIC

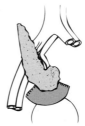

Typical outcomes
1 yr graft survival 75%

- Typical indications
  - Diabetes
- Technical notes
  - Pancreas and duodenum implanted into iliac fossa
  - Often with simultaneous kindey transplant
- Typical complications
  - Pancreatitis
  - Acute rejection
  - Vascular thrombosis

SMALL BOWEL

Typical outcomes
1 yr graft survival 60%

- Typical indications
  - Short bowel due to resection/ vascular accident
  - Congenital atresia
- Typical complications
  - Acute rejection
  - GVHD

Definitions

Transplantation is the removal of an organ or tissue from one organism and its surgical implantation into another organism to provide structure and/or function. A *graft* is the organ or tissue transplanted. *Allografting* (also known as *homografting*) is transplantation between organisms of the same species (i.e. human to human). *Xenografting* is transplantation between organisms of different species (e.g. pig to human). Grafts may be placed in the same ('correct') anatomical location (*orthotopic* transplantation; e.g. heart transplant) or in a non-anatomical (*heterotopic* transplantation; e.g. kidney transplant). The graft comes from a *donor* and is implanted into a *recipient*. Donors may be *cadaveric* (usually brainstem death victims if human), *living related* (LRD) (family members sharing large genetic elements with the recipient) or *living unrelated* (LURD) (altruistic individuals donating one of a pair of organs).

Key points

- All but identical twin transplants require immunosuppression.
- Graft rejection can be hyperacute, acute or chronic.
- Long-term immunosuppression causes diseases in its own right.
- Kidney, pancreas, liver, heart and lung transplantation are well established with high success rates. Small bowel transplantation is being progressively developed.

Immunology of transplantation

- Pre-existing cell surface antigens (e.g. ABO and related blood groups) stimulate pre-existing humoral immunity in the form of antibodies. All grafts must be ABO-matched or hyperacute rejection will occur.
- Class 1 MHC antigens (e.g. HLA-A, HLA-B, HLA-C) exist on nucleated cell surfaces and stimulate activation of recipient CD8 positive (cytotoxic) T lymphocytes. Optimizing Class 1 matching reduces the risk of acute rejection episodes.
- Class 2 MHC antigens (e.g. DR, DP, DQ) are found on cells such as macrophages, monocytes and B lymphocytes and stimulate CD4 positive (helper) T lymphocytes. Optimizing Class 2 matching reduces the risk of mixed humoral/cell-mediated rejection.

Graft rejection

- Hyperacute rejection—occurs shortly after graft enters host circulation. Caused by preformed antibody recognition of cell surface antigens and can be largely prevented by crossmatching between recipient serum and donor cells.
- Acute rejection—can occur at any time if the life of a graft but is most common in the first months after transplantation. Caused by cell-mediated immunity against HLA antigens. May be reduced or prevented by immunosuppression.
- Chronic rejection—occurs after months and years. Causes may be multifaoctorial including low grade cell-mediated attack due to HLA mismatching, chronic infection, underlying organ disease.

Immunosuppression

- All immunosuppressives result in non-specific suppression of immune defence and increase the life time risk of infection and certain malignancies for the recipient.
- Typical infections under immunosuppression include; CMV, herpes group viruses, *Pneumocystis*, *Candida*, *Aspergilla*, *Cryptococcus*.
- Typical malignancies under immunosuppression include; BCC skin, SCC skin, B-cell lymphomas.

Drug group	Effect	Side-effects
Corticosteroids	Suppress all inflammatory elements of the immune response	'Cushingoid' effects
Antiproliferatives (methotrexate, azathioprine, mycophenolate)	Prevent cell-mediated cell mitosis and amplification of response	Renal and hepatic dysfunction, marrow suppression
Calcineurin blockade (ciclosporin, tacrolimus)	Suppress T cells and rescue IL-2 release	Nephrotoxicity
Biological effectors (antilymphocyte globulin, OKT3 anti-CD3 Ab, anti CD5 Ab)	Block specific parts of the immune responses	Fevers, nausea, vomiting, myalgia

Graft-versus-host disease

- Caused by donor immune cells present in the graft mounting immunological attack on recipient tissues.
- Causes skin, liver and lung inflammation.
- May be reduced by perfusing the graft thoroughly prior to implantation to 'wash-out' donor lymphocytes.

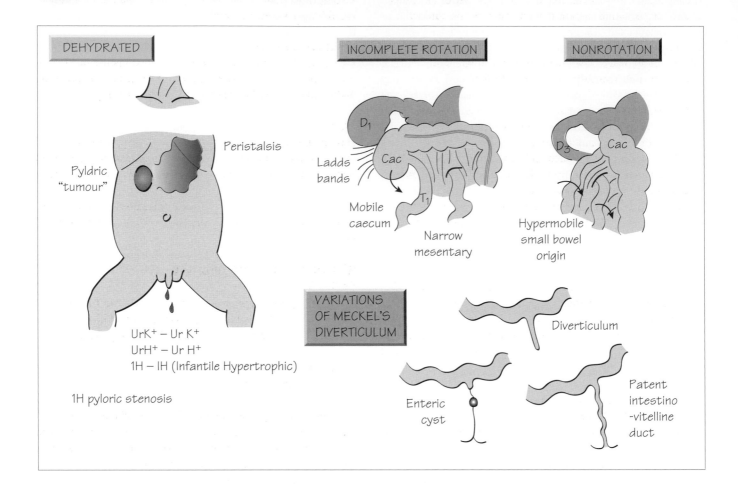

DEHYDRATED

Peristalsis

Pyldric "tumour"

UrK⁺ – Ur K⁺
UrH⁺ – Ur H⁺
1H – IH (Infantile Hypertrophic)

1H pyloric stenosis

INCOMPLETE ROTATION

D_1

Ladds bands

Cac

Mobile caecum

T_1

Narrow mesentary

NONROTATION

D_3 Cac

Hypermobile small bowel origin

VARIATIONS OF MECKEL'S DIVERTICULUM

Diverticulum

Enteric cyst

Patent intestino-vitelline duct

Infantile hypertrophic pyloric stenosis
Definition
This is a condition characterized by hypertrophy of the circular muscle of the gastric pylorus that obstructs gastric outflow.

Aetiology
The aetiology is unknown but it affects 1 in 450 children; 85% male, often firstborn; 20% have family history.

Clinical features
• Non-bile-stained, projectile vomiting (after feeds) beginning at 2–6 weeks. May be bloodstained.
• Baby is hungry, constipated and dehydrated. Loss of H^+ and Cl^- from stomach and K^+ from kidney causes hypochloraemic, hypokalaemic metabolic alkalosis.
• Palpable pyloric 'tumour' during a test feed or after vomiting.
• Gastric peristalsis may be seen. Ultrasound confirms the diagnosis.

Management
• Correct dehydration and electrolyte imbalance with 0.45% NaCl in dextrose 5% with added K^+. May take 24–48 hours to become normal.
• Ramstedt's pyloromyotomy via transverse RUQ or per umbilical incision or laparoscopically. Normal feeding can commence within 24 hours.

Malrotation of the gut
Definition and aetiology
'Malrotation' is often used to describe a number of conditions (1 in 500 live births) that are caused by failure of the intestine to rotate into the correct anatomical position during embryological development. Most common types are incomplete rotation and non-rotation.
Complications that can result include:
• Volvulus (leading to risk of bowel necrosis); usually small bowel ± caecum/proximal colon.
• Internal herniation (via abnormally large paraduodenal recesses and paracolic spaces).

• Duodenal obstruction (usually incomplete and intermittent); often said to be due to Ladd's bands (peritoneal tissue related to incomplete rotation) but probably due to rotation of a narrow small bowel mesenteric origin.

Clinical features
Bile-stained vomiting in the newborn period is the most common presentation but older children may present with recurrent abdominal pain, abdominal distension and vomiting.

Management
• If diagnosed prior to acute presentation: surgery to 'complete' the non-rotation; placing the colon in the left abdomen and small bowel to the right (widening the mesenertic attachment with fixation).
• Acute presentations: release the obstructions, resect non-viable bowel ± fixation of the bowel in normal anatomical position.

Meckel's diverticulum
Definition
Meckel's diverticulum is the remnant of the vitello-intestinal duct forming a blind-ending pouch on the antimesenteric border of the terminal ileum and is present in 2% of the population.

Clinical features
Most are asymptomatic.
  May present with:
• Rectal bleeding (often due to ulceration of the normal ileal mucosa opposite the diverticulum due to acid secreting (gastric antral type) epithelium within the diverticulum—detectable by technetium pertechnate scan in 70% of cases.
• 'Appendicitis' (Meckel's diverticulitis).
• Acute ileoileal intussusception.
• Volvulus (due to intestine-vityelline band/duct with small bowel rotation around it).

Management
Surgical excision, even if found incidentally.

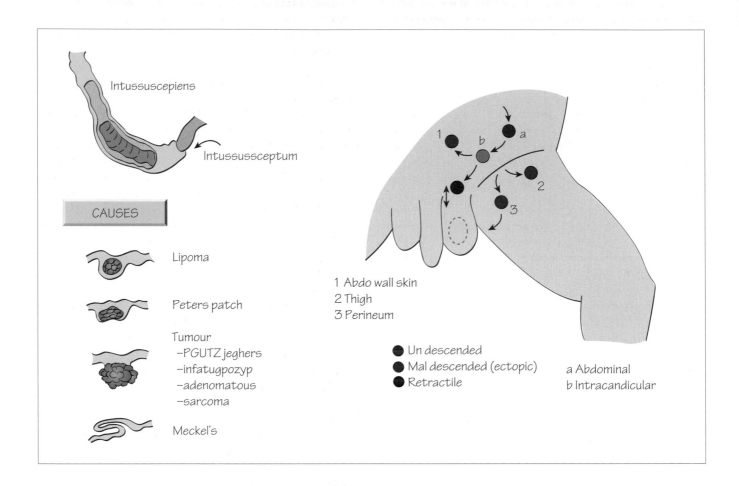

Intussuscepiens

Intussussceptum

CAUSES

Lipoma

Peters patch

Tumour
 –PGUTZ jeghers
 –infatugpozyp
 –adenomatous
 –sarcoma

Meckel's

1 Abdo wall skin
2 Thigh
3 Perineum

● Un descended
● Mal descended (ectopic)
● Retractile

a Abdominal
b Intracandicular

Gastro-oesophageal reflux

Definition
This is a common condition characterized by incompetence of the LOS, resulting in retrograde passage of gastric contents into the oesophagus, leading to vomiting.

Aetiology
Transient LOS relaxation caused by:
• Increased volumes in feeds overwhelming gastric capacity.
• 'Slumped' seating position.

Clinical features
• Vomiting, usually bile-stained, not related to feeds, may contain blood (indicates oesophagitis) and rarely is projectile.
• Respiratory symptoms are frequently present of often caused by microaspiration of gastric content.

• Apnoea, stridor, wheezing, chronic (nocturnal) cough and failure to thrive may all be present.

Investigations
Most cases require no investigations and the diagnosis and treatment can be based on clinical features. If oesophagitis, stricture, anaemia or aspiration is suspected, a barium swallow, gastric scintigraphy (good for diagnosis of pulmonary aspiration), oesophagoscopy and biopsy, 24-hour pH monitoring and oesophageal manometry are indicated.

Treatment
As there is a natural tendency towards spontaneous improvement with age (most have resolved by age 18 months), a conservative approach is adopted initially: smaller, thicker feeds, positioning infant in 30° head-up prone position after feeds,

antacids, H_2 receptor blockers, proton pump inhibitors ± prokinetic agents.

Surgery (laparoscopic Nissen fundoplication) is reserved for failure for respond to conservative treatment with oesophageal stricture or severe pulmonary aspiration.

Intussusception
Definitions
Intussusception is the invagination of one segment of bowel into an adjacent distal segment. The segment that invaginates is called the *intussusceptum* and the segment into which it invaginates the *intussuscepiens*. The tip of the intussusceptum is called the *apex* or *lead point*.

Aetiology
• 90% are idiopathic.
• Viral infection can lead to hyperplasia of Peyer's patches which become the apex of an intussusception.
• Other lead points include Meckel's diverticulum, a polyp or a duplication cyst.

Clinical features
• Most common cause of intestinal obstruction in infants 3–12 months. Males > females.
• Presents with pain (attacks of colicky pain every 15–20 minutes, lasting 2–3 minutes with screaming and drawing up of legs), pallor, vomiting and lethargy between attacks.
• Sausage-shaped mass in RUQ, empty RIF (sign de Dance).
• Passage of blood and mucus ('redcurrant jelly' stool).
• Tachycardia and dehydration.

Diagnosis
• Plain X-ray may show intestinal obstruction and sometimes the outline of the intussusception.
• Ultrasonography may help showing RUQ mass.
• Definite diagnosis by air or (less common) barium enema.

Management
• IV fluids to resuscitate infant (shock is frequent because of fluid sequesteration in the bowel).
• Air or barium reduction of intussusception if no peritonitis (75% of cases).
• Remainder require surgical reduction.

Inguinoscrotal conditions
Acute scrotum
Definition
The *acute scrotum* is a red, swollen, painful scrotum caused by torsion of the hydatid of Morgagni (60%), torsion of the testis (30%), epididymo-orchitis (10%) and idiopathic scrotal oedema (10%).

Management
• All cases of 'acute scrotum' should be explored.
• If true testicular torsion, treatment is bilateral orchidopexy (orchidectomy of affected testis if gangrenous).
• If torsion is hydatid of Morgagni, treatment is removal of hydatid on affected side only.

Inguinal hernia and hydrocele
Definitions and aetiology
During the seventh month of gestation the testis descends from the posterior abdominal wall into the scrotum through a peritoneal diverticulum called the *processus vaginalis*, which obliterates just before birth. An *inguinal hernia* in an infant is a swelling in the inguinal area due to failure of obliteration of the processus vaginalis, allowing bowel (rarely omentum) to descend within the hernial sac below the external inguinal ring. A *hydrocele* is a collection of fluid around the testis that has trickled down from the peritoneal cavity via a narrow, but patent, processus vaginalis.

Diagnosis
• Diagnosis of a hydrocele is usually obvious: the scrotum contains fluid and transilluminates brilliantly.
• Diagnosis of a hernia may be entirely on the mother's given history or a lump may be obvious.
• Strangulation is a serious complication as it may compromise bowel and/or the blood supply to the testis.

Management
Both hernia and hydrocele should be treated by operation to obliterate the remaining processus vaginalis.

Undescended testis
Definitions and aetiology
A *congenital undescended testis* (UDT) is one that has not reached the bottom of the scrotum at 3 months post-term. A *retractile testis* is one that can be manipulated to the bottom of the scrotum. An *ectopic testis* is one that has strayed from the normal path of descent.

Diagnosis
Most UDTs are found at the superficial inguinal pouch and associated with hypoplastic hemi-scrotum and inguinal hernia.

Management
• Treatment is by orchidopexy and should be performed at 6–12 months.
• UDTs are at increased risk of developing malignancy, even after orchidopexy and require long-term surveillance.

Index

Page numbers in *italics* refer to illustrations.

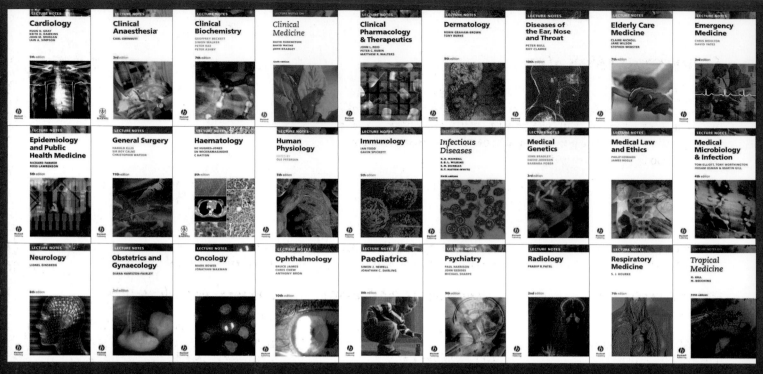
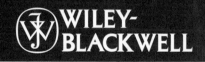
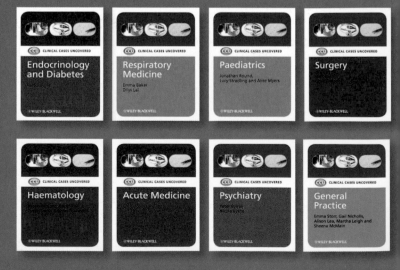